COPING WITH ECZEMA

DR ROBERT YOUNGSON, MB, ChB, DTM&H, DO, FRC Ophth, a former medical consultant, is now a full-time writer. He is the author of twenty-one popular medical and science books including *Coping Successfully with Hay Fever* and *Living with Asthma* (both Sheldon Press 1995) and has also written extensively on medical topics for *Reader's Digest* and *Good Housekeeping* books. He has made many radio broadcasts and has appeared on television.

Overcoming Common Problems Series

For a full list of titles please contact
Sheldon Press, Marylebone Road, London NW1 4DU

The Assestiveness Workbook
A plan for busy women
JOANNA GUTMANN

Birth Over Thirty
SHEILA KITZINGER

Body Language
How to read others' thoughts by their
gestures
ALLAN PEASE

Body Language in Relationships
DAVID COHEN

Calm Down
How to cope with frustration and anger
DR PAUL HAUCK

Changing Course
How to take charge of your career
SUE DYSON AND STEPHEN HOARE

Comfort for Depression
JANET HORWOOD

Coping Successfully with Agoraphobia
DR KENNETH HAMBLY

Coping Successfully with Migraine
SUE DYSON

Coping Successfully with Pain
NEVILLE SHONE

Coping Successfully with Panic Attacks
SHIRLEY TRICKETT

Coping Successfully with Prostate Problems
ROSY REYNOLDS

**Coping Successfully with Your Hyperactive
Child**
DR PAUL CARSON

Coping Successfully with Your Irritable Bowel
ROSEMARY NICOL

Coping Successfully with Your Second Child
FIONA MARSHALL

Coping with Anxiety and Depression
SHIRLEY TRICKETT

Coping with Blushing
DR ROBERT EDELMANN

Coping with Cot Death
SARAH MURPHY

Coping with Depression and Elation
DR PATRICK McKEON

Coping with Strokes
DR TOM SMITH

Coping with Suicide
DR DONALD SCOTT

Coping with Thrush
CAROLINE CLAYTON

Curing Arthritis – The Drug-Free Way
MARGARET HILLS

Curing Arthritis
More ways to a drug-free life
MARGARET HILLS

Curing Arthritis Diet Book
MARGARET HILLS

**Curing Coughs, Colds and Flu – The Drug-
Free Way**
MARGARET HILLS

Curing Illness – The Drug-Free Way
MARGARET HILLS

Depression
DR PAUL HAUCK

Divorce and Separation
Every woman's guide to a new life
ANGELA WILLIAMS

Don't Blame Me!
How to stop blaming yourself and other people
TONY GOUGH

Everything You Need to Know about Shingles
DR ROBERT YOUNGSON

Family First Aid and Emergency Handbook
DR ANDREW SRANWAY

Overcoming Common Problems Series

Overcoming Common Problems Series

Overcoming Common Problems

COPING WITH ECZEMA

Dr Robert Youngson

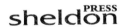

First published in Great Britain in 1995 by
Sheldon Press, SPCK, Marylebone Road, London NW1 4DU

British Library Cataloguing-in-Publication Data
A catalogue record for this book is available from the British Library

ISBN 0–85969–736–3

Photoset by Deltatype Ltd, Ellesmere Port, Cheshire
Printed in Great Britain by Biddles Ltd, Guildford and King's Lynn

To Eric

Contents

Introduction

At one time doctors used the term 'eczema' to describe skin inflammation for which there was no known cause. When there *was* a recognizable external cause, the condition was called 'dermatitis' even if the appearances and other clinical features were exactly the same. Eczema was considered to be caused by some mysterious constitutional factor, particular to the individual. It was said to be an endogenous condition (from Greek *endo*, meaning 'inside', and *geneos*, meaning 'origin'). Dermatitis was considered to be exogenous (from Greek *exo*, outside) and to be caused exclusively by the external factor, whatever its nature. Recent advances in our understanding of how skin disorders come about have shown that this distinction is artificial and can no longer be maintained.

We now understand that *all* cases of persistent, itchy skin rash of the eczema type are brought about by both internal and external factors. Enormous advances have been made in the understanding of these factors and the purpose of this book is to explain them to you so that you will have a reliable factual basis for coping with the problem. If you read this book with care, the chances are that you will know at least as much about eczema as the average doctor. Even in general textbooks of skin disease (dermatology), the amount of information available on eczema is often less than is contained in this book. Once you have grasped the scientific facts behind eczema, you will be in a position to understand the medical treatment of the condition. This, too, is fully explained.

No book of this or any other kind can ever be an adequate substitute for a consultation with a doctor. Every person suffering from eczema, however mild the condition, should have the benefit of medical consultation. But if you have studied this book you will be much better placed to discuss the subject intelligently, to understand what the doctor tells you, and even, perhaps, to put some searching questions.

There is a considerable amount of detail in this book, and nearly all of it fits together into a logical framework which I hope you will be

1

able to follow fairly easily. To help you to do this I have included a number of short case histories of patients. These histories, in which the names and background details have been fictionalized, will help to make a number of important points. They will also, I hope, help to keep you reading. There is nothing like a bit of human interest to lighten the burden of study.

1

What is Eczema?

The word 'eczema', with its strange and unique spelling, would seem to imply some great medical mystery. In fact, the term is purely descriptive and comes from the Greek words *ek-*, meaning 'out' and *zein*, meaning 'to boil'. The Greeks actually used the word *ekzema* for skin eruptions but probably applied it to a wider range of skin conditions than we do today. An early English reference, of 1753, stated that eczema was 'a name given by the ancient physicians, to any fiery pustule on the skin'.

Today, the term is used for a persistent, itchy skin disorder that may progress to tiny blisters, known as vesicles, which may leak a watery fluid that forms crusts. The most striking feature of eczema is its constant tendency to itch. This leads to scratching and this, in turn, causes damage to the skin in the form of surface hardening, thickening and a whitish scaling known as lichenification. This, again, is a purely descriptive word implying a (rather fanciful) resemblance to the spread of lichen on rock.

Eczema is most prevalent in infancy and childhood and fewer cases are found during the period of puberty and adolescence. The condition, however, often persists into adult life. Rarely – in less than 2 per cent of cases – eczema appears for the first time in people over 45 years of age.

The types of eczema

First, to clear up any confusion, an explanation of the term 'dermatitis'. Dermatitis is not, as is commonly thought, a disease. The word simply means 'inflammation of the skin'. *Derma* is Greek for 'skin, hide or leather', and *-itis* is the common Greek ending meaning 'inflammation of'. The term is thus correctly applied to any one of the many hundreds of skin disorders that feature redness, discomfort, heat and swelling – the classical signs (*rubor, dolor, calor* and *tumor*) of inflammation. But to call a condition dermatitis is to say nothing more about it than that it is a skin inflammation. If we want to say more, we must put another word before 'dermatitis'.

Many dermatologists insist that the term 'eczema' also simply means 'inflammation of the skin' and the terms 'dermatitis' and 'eczema' are interchangeable. Those who take this view also hold, quite logically, that eczema is not a disease and that if we wish to use the term to refer to anything more than skin inflammation it must be qualified by another word placed before it. The term 'eczema' is, however, so well established and so universally applied to a well-recognized clinical condition that the purists are probably fighting a losing battle. If we use the term with a clear understanding of the type of eczema to which we are referring (see below), we will not go far wrong.

Although all forms of eczema result from the same basic processes and are essentially similar, it is convenient to divide them into two large categories – a group in which there is a strong hereditary element but no obvious external cause, known as atopic eczema or atopic dermatitis, and a group which is not hereditary and in which there are often obvious external causes. Atopic eczema is essentially a disorder of the immune system and is an allergic condition. The same immune system process can cause hay fever and asthma, which are also atopic conditions. These other manifestations of atopy are fully covered in two other Sheldon Press books, *Living with Asthma* and *Coping Successfully with Hay Fever*.

The principles underlying atopic, or allergic, eczema are central to an understanding of *all* forms of eczema, and for this reason chapter 3 – *Understanding Atopic Eczema* – is the most important in the book. That chapter outlines the very recent knowledge of the genetic basis of atopy and deals with the processes in the immune system that lead to the abnormalities in the skin which occur in all forms of eczema. Chapter 5 is concerned with those forms of eczema that are not primarily hereditary in orgin.

How common is eczema?

It is difficult to get precise information on this. Different surveys have given figures ranging from 0.7 per cent to as high as 20 per cent. These differences probably arise from differing definitions of the degree of severity of cases that should be included, and differences in the way the data are obtained. But there is no doubt that eczema is very common and that it is getting commoner. One series on the occurrences (the epidemiology) of atopic eczema showed that, in developed countries, 1.4 to 3.1 per cent of those born before 1960 had some degree of eczema, while 8.9 to 20.4 per cent of those born after 1970 had the disease. This is an extraordinary rise. There has been some controversy as to the reason for this increase in the prevalence of atopic dermatitis, but it is generally attributed to such factors as:

- rising levels of environmental irritant pollution;
- airborne substances promoting allergy (allergens) such as house dust mite excreta, animal saliva, animal skin scales (dander) and grass and tree pollens;
- infections;
- food allergy.

We now know that in a person who is genetically predisposed, environmental stimuli trigger off eczema. This is fully discussed in chapter 3.

Associated conditions

About half of all the people with atopic eczema also have hay fever or asthma or both. And in about three quarters of cases another member of the family has eczema, asthma or hay fever or a combination of these. The reason for this close association of the three conditions is now well understood. It is that there is an underlying condition that predisposes the person to any or all of the three disorders. This condition is known as atopy.

Fortunately, in the majority of cases eczema is worst in early childhood and tends to get better gradually with time. In many cases, indeed, the disease clears up altogether between the ages of two and five years. However, it is important to understand that, even if this happens, the person concerned remains especially liable, throughout the whole of life, to develop eczema as a result of contact with both physical and chemical irritants. This vulnerability is one of the reasons why people with eczema cannot be divided in a clear-cut way into endogenous and exogenous cases. Unfortunately, it can also have a serious effect on the range of suitable employment.

Here is a typical case history of uncomplicated infantile eczema.

CASE HISTORY
Bernard – an only child and a late arrival – is his parents' pride and joy. But they are horrified to find that his beautiful smooth skin has become disfigured by a rash . . .

PERSONAL DETAILS
Name Bernard Hughes
Age 4 months
Occupation N/A
Family Parents alive and well; no siblings.

MEDICAL BACKGROUND
Bernard's parents married late and tried for a child for nearly five years. Bernard is a lovely, healthy child who has given very little trouble with crying or sleeplessness. He has had no particular teething problems and no history of feeding difficulties or intestinal upset. Mr and Mrs Hughes are both reasonably healthy apart from the fact that Mr Hughes suffers from fairly severe asthma which he keeps under control with regular use of inhalers.

THE PRESENT COMPLAINT
Both of Bernard's parents attend when he is brought to their GP's surgery – a circumstance that alerts the doctor to the level of their concern. Mr and Mrs Hughes are horrified to find that Bernard has developed an area of greasy, yellowish scales on the top of his head. Below the scales, and in the scalp around the affected area, the skin is obviously inflamed. Bernard also has some flakiness in and around his eyebrows.

THE CONSULTATION
The doctor checks that Bernard's previous health has been good and that he is feeding and sleeping well and gaining weight

normally. She asks Mrs Hughes to undress Bernard and checks over the whole skin area. Only the scalp and the eyebrows are affected. After examining the rash carefully with a hand lens the doctor informs Mr and Mrs Hughes that Bernard has a mild condition known as 'cradle cap'. Medically, it is known as seborrhoeic dermatitis.

This diagnosis frightens the parents and the doctor has difficulty in reassuring them that it is an unimportant and usually self-limiting condition. Mrs Hughes is most anxious to be reassured that this is not a form of eczema but the doctor is non-committal. She is aware of the father's history of asthma and recognizes the possibility that Bernard may have inherited atopy. She recommends that the scalp scales should be softened each evening with olive oil or liquid paraffin and gently brushed off in the mornings. No other treatment is needed.

THE SECOND CONSULTATION
Bernard's parents attend again four months later, this time demanding urgent action. Bernard has developed a red, scaly rash with small blisters, on his scalp, face, hands and around the creases of his elbows and knees. The rash is obviously intensely itchy as he is constantly trying to rub or scratch it. His sleep is being disturbed and, for the first time, he is keeping his parents awake at night. The parents insist on knowing what the condition is and are seriously distressed when the doctor confirms that Bernard has infantile eczema. The doctor assures them that it is most uncommon for the face to continue to be affected and that the facial eczema should soon clear up.

THE FOLLOW-UP
The doctor is relieved to find that her prediction is realized. The rash on Bernard's face disappears completely within two months leaving the skin unblemished. Unfortunately, the rash on his limbs persists and occasionally becomes so severe that the doctor is forced to prescribe hydrocortisone cream. This is used in minimal amounts, however, and the doctor assures the parents that there are no side effects from such treatment.

WHAT IS ECZEMA?

For a few years, Bernard continues to suffer the itchy rash, but this gradually becomes, on average, less obvious and, to his parents' delight, it clears up completely before his fifth birthday. The doctor explains that this is quite characteristic of infantile eczema and that, although she cannot guarantee that the trouble will not recur, she thinks this is unlikely.

2

All About the Skin

There is far more to eczema than just the changes in the skin described in the next chapter. But from the point of view of the sufferer, it is the skin changes that matter. To understand these you must first have some idea of the nature, structure and function of normal skin. It makes a lot of sense for anyone with a skin problem or anyone responsible for a child with eczema to know as much as possible about the skin.

Some facts about the skin

There are some very odd ideas around concerning the skin. I have heard people suggest, for instance, that the skin can be split into seven layers. Others have it that the skin is adversely affected by eating lots of chocolate or that you can sweat out poisons from the body through the skin. Let's forget these stories and get down to some real facts.

The skin is much more than just a passive waterproof cover for the body. Because it is constantly being stretched, compressed, bent, stood upon, rubbed, poked and scratched, it has to be flexible and tough and have the ability to repair itself rapidly after injury. These properties of the skin are, to a greater or lesser degree, impaired by skin disease such as eczema. Doctors, especially skin specialists (dermatologists) think of the skin as one of the body organs, to be classed with other body organs such as the kidneys, lungs and intestines. It is certainly a living, vital structure although covered with a thin layer of dead cells and, being exposed, it is constantly at risk of injury. Life is impossible without the skin; until comparatively recently, people who suffered more than 30 per cent burns usually died from loss of fluid, but major developments in the management of severe burns and fluid replacement have changed all this. The fact, however, emphasizes one of the most important functions of healthy skin – to retain body fluid.

The skin is the largest organ of the body, ranging in area, in adults, from 15,000 to 20,000 square centimetres (16 to 20 square feet).

9

Under normal conditions it is self-renewing and self-repairing. It acts as a heat-regulating mechanism for the body and provides a remarkable degree of protection from the outside world. It is exquisitely sensitive to touch, pressure, pain, irritation, heat and cold. A great deal of essential information from the outside world enters the body by way of the skin and is conveyed to the brain. If you are sitting in a chair as you read this, or standing in a bookshop wondering whether to buy this book, special nerve endings in the skin of your bottom or your feet are firing off messages to your brain informing it of the pressure.

In addition to preventing undue loss of water – the interior of the body is largely watery – the skin controls the extent to which certain soluble substances in the blood (electrolytes) are lost or retained. It does the same for certain proteins. If you exert yourself enough in hot conditions, however, you can lose remarkable quantities of water – up to about six litres a day – in the form of sweat. This is more than the total volume of the blood. Such losses are, of course, rapidly fatal unless the fluid is replaced by drinking. The evaporation of water from a surface removes considerable quantities of heat from the surface. This is one of the ways in which the skin controls body temperature. Flushing of the skin, by a widening of its blood vessels, also helps to cool the body. In cold conditions, the skin blood vessels close down so that the amount of heat passing through the skin is greatly reduced and heat is conserved.

The skin screens against light damage by absorbing light energy into the pigment melanin. This pigment is contained in cells called melanocytes that lie below the surface and largely determine the skin colour. If the melanocytes have many melanin granules, the skin is dark, if not, it is light-coloured. The skin is also a complete barrier against the alpha particles of radioactivity and is only just penetrated by beta particles. Gamma rays, however, pass right through the body.

Healthy skin provides considerable resistance to attack by germs. This is partly because it contains immune system cells that attack germs and partly because the skin is constantly shedding the flat, surface, dead cells of its outer layer (see below). This constant shedding of skin scales actively dislodges germs. The skin synthesizes vitamin D under the influence of sunlight.

Skin pores are the small openings in the skin through which the sweat passes from tiny glands situated in the deepest layers of the skin or just under it. Other pores in the skin are the hair follicles into which open the sebaceous glands producing the oily secretion sebum. In the skin of the nose, the hairs in these follicles are usually small in comparison with the sebaceous glands, so that the pores appear to be concerned solely with sebum production.

The structure of the skin

The skin varies considerably in thickness in different parts of the body. Eyelid skin is only about half a millimetre thick, while the skin on the soles of the feet and the palms of the hand is often 4 millimetres thick. Skin has two layers – the inner corium, or dermis, also known as the 'true skin', and the outer epidermis.

The epidermis

As its name implies, this layer lies beyond or outside the true skin. The epidermis is structurally simple with no nerves, blood vessels, or hair follicles, and much of it acts as a rapidly replaceable surface capable of tolerating much abrasion and trauma. The outermost cells of the epidermis are dead and are continuously shed, being replaced by cells derived from the lower, living, part. On average, it takes about 30 days from the time a cell is produced at the bottom of the epidermis to the time it is shed from the surface. An adult sheds about nine grams of epidermal scales every day. Most of the growth and reproduction of the underlying cells occurs during the night when we are asleep.

The deepest layer of the epidermis, from which all the other epidermal cells derive, is called the basal cell layer. This layer contains the pigment melanin in granules in the melanocytes. When cells of the basal cell layer become cancerous they produce the common skin cancer known as a basal cell carcinoma or rodent ulcer. If you must get cancer, this is the one to pick. It never spreads remotely and, treated reasonably early, has a 100 per cent cure rate. Between the basal cell layer and the dead outer cells is the prickle cell layer, so called because the cells look a bit like holly leaves. When a local group of prickle cells grow abnormally fast you have a wart. Prickle cells are prompted to do so by viruses of the human papillomavirus family.

The main function of the prickle cells is to make a tough, insoluble protein called keratin. As the prickle cells are pushed towards the surface by the growth of other cells below them, they gradually die, losing their DNA nuclei and becoming little more than flat envelopes containing keratin. The thickness of the keratin layer at any point on the skin depends on what you do with that bit of skin. If you treat it gently, the layer of dead cells will be quite thin. But if you constantly press on it, as when using a pick and shovel or wearing excessively tight shoes, the keratin layer will greatly thicken to form a 'corn' or callus. Doctors often refer to the keratin layer as the layer of cornified cells, and, incidentally, fingernails and hair are mainly made from keratin.

Scattered throughout the basal and prickle cells are many living cells, of a quite different type, called Langerhans cells. These are active cells capable of eating up germs, skin debris and other unwanted things. Like all 'eating' cells they are called phagocytes. This word comes from the Greek *phagos*, meaning 'eating' and *kutos*, a 'container or hollow vessel'. The Langerhans cells have long, branching arms and are a good deal larger than the general run of phagocytes, so they are called macrophages – which just means 'big eaters'. We have known for some time that macrophages are cells of the immune system. Recent research has shown that the Langerhans cells are very important in bringing about the damage that is a feature of eczema. They do this by providing a recognition system for substances to which the person is allergic. These are called antigens. If Langerhens cells are in short supply, allergic contact dermatitis *does not occur*.

The dermis

The dermis, which lies on a layer of fat, is structurally more complicated than the epidermis. Its outer surface – the surface that is in contact with the basal cell layer of the epidermis – is not flat but is thrown up into millions of tiny hillocks, called papillae, each of which contains a minute collection of blood vessels. When surgeons are taking split skin grafts to cover raw areas they cut the skin at such a level that the blade slices through the tips of these little papillae. So when the cut is just right, the cut surface shows thousands of tiny red spots. This rich blood supply allows the skin to control body temperature and provides for rapid healing of cuts and wounds.

The papillae are not scattered randomly, but are arranged in double rows which form a pattern of slightly raised, straight or curved ridges in the epidermis. The pattern is unique to the individual and the particular pattern on the pads of the fingers produces the fingerprints by which people can be identified. Even identical twins have different patterns of papillary ridges.

The dermis consists of a felted meshwork of fibrous and elastic tissue, through which pass the hair follicles in which the hairs are growing and the ducts of the sweat glands. Each hair follicle has a tiny muscle attached to it in the dermis. When this muscle tightens the hair follicle, which normally lies at an angle, is pulled into an upright position. As a result, the hair 'stands on end'. These muscles, known as the arrector pili muscles, contract when we are frightened. Their contraction also pulls down the skin around the exit region of the hair shaft, causing 'goose-pimples'.

The bulbs of the hair follicles and the main, coiled bodies of the sweat glands lie in the fatty tissue under the dermis. The average person has about two million sweat glands and, when not exerting, loses about a pint of sweat a day.

Scattered throughout the dermis, at various levels, are millions of tiny specialized nerve endings providing sensitivity to many kinds of stimuli – light and firm touch, pressure, pain, and high and low temperatures.

Other general points

Some of the skin nerves are capable of responding to the most subtle stimuli, such as those caused by the delicate touch of a tiny moving insect. The response to such a stimulus will often be to produce the sensation of itching and evoke an almost automatic scratch reflex. The same effect is produced on these nerves by the release of certain irritating substances actually *within* the substance of the skin. This is a very important feature of eczema.

ALL ABOUT THE SKIN

Because the skin is the only visible organ of the body we are, naturally, sensitive to its appearance. It is, in short, an organ of sexual attraction, and male and female skins differ considerably in appearance. This is partly because hormones such as oestrogen and testosterone have a considerable effect on the skin, controlling and promoting hair growth according to the sex. There are several conditions in which abnormal amounts of the wrong hormone can cause women's skin to resemble that of men, and vice versa.

Sexual attraction, determined only partly by fashion, decrees that skin should be smooth and free from blemish. Excess oiliness is usually considered undesirable in the West, and white-skinned people will often apply powder to the skin to improve the appearance. On the other hand, black skin can appear too powdery in the absence of adequate sebaceous secretion. In some cultures, decoration of the skin by tattooing or stretching are considered sexually attractive.

The perceived value of a suntan varies from area to area and from time to time. People with dark-coloured skins will often prefer to be lightened; those with white skins will often prefer to be darkened. By now, everyone should be aware that undue exposure of white skins to sunlight is undesirable. Sunlight contains ultraviolet light (UVL) and this is the cause of sunburning. But UVL has other effects and these are cumulative. If, over a period, you get more than a minimal total dose, it will damage a protein in the dermis, called collagen. This protein keeps the skin tight and elastic. As a result of collagen damage, your skin either stretches and hangs in folds, or becomes excessively wrinkled and old-looking. Both may happen. This kind of disfigurement is a common fate of white people living in the tropics and of long-term sun-worshippers who take every opportunity to sunbathe. The indigenous people in tropical areas are protected by plenty of melanin pigment that acts as a sun-screen. Even in the tropics, white people who are protected from the sun suffer no ill effects and their skin remains smooth and elastic.

Ultraviolet light also damages the DNA in the deeper, living cells of the skin. This can cause a condition known as solar keratosis in which scaly, coloured, white patches form that can progress to a type of skin cancer called squamous cell carcinoma. Much more commonly, ultraviolet light causes the less serious skin cancer basal cell carcinoma or rodent ulcer, already mentioned. Most seriously of all, ultraviolet light DNA damage can lead to malignant melanoma. This is not particularly common, but is getting commoner and is very nasty indeed.

With this background knowledge of the structure and properties of the skin, you are now well equipped to proceed to a study of the disease process known as eczema. The next chapter is the most difficult of the book but because it involves a look at genetics and the functioning of the immune system, is also the most interesting. After chapter 3 it is all plain sailing.

3

Understanding Atopic Eczema

It has been obvious for many years that eczema has a hereditary basis. An interesting Danish study of eczema involving 812 pairs of twins showed that, in identical twins, when one twin had eczema, the other also had it in 72 per cent of cases. When non-identical twins were checked, it was found that eczema in one was paired with eczema in the other in only 23 per cent of cases. This is impressive evidence that a genetic element is operating.

Many families feature the condition, often in one generation after another. In many cases, several members of the family are affected. It has also long been known that eczema is associated with asthma and with hay fever. Many families in which one of these conditions regularly appears will also have people suffering from one or two of the others. The reason for this seemingly improbable association of hereditary conditions has, until recently, been a complete mystery. Happily, new facts arising from recent research have thrown light on the mystery. As we shall see, it has recently been established that the tendency to eczema and to these other conditions is inherited through several genes.

It is important to understand that eczema is not inherited in the sense that diseases like sickle cell disease, haemophilia or cystic fibrosis are inherited. If the full gene pattern for these conditions is present, the disease will appear. In the case of eczema, what is inherited is a particular state which makes people much more prone than normal to develop eczema or asthma or hay fever. This state is called atopy.

Atopy is a strange word derived from the Greek *atopos*, meaning 'unusual'. This, in turn comes from the Greek roots *a-*, meaning 'not' and *topos*, meaning 'a place'. The word was originally used to mean simply 'out of place'. But in 1923 a scientist called A. F. Coca, writing in the *Journal of Immunology*, described how he needed a word to describe a tendency to abnormal hypersensitivity caused by genetic influences. The word had to reflect the fact that contact with one part of the body could produce an effect elsewhere in the body. At a loss, he consulted Professor Edward D. Perry, who suggested the word 'atopy'. This was appropriate as atopy can manifest itself in various unexpected parts of the body.

What is atopy?

This question cannot be answered all at once, because the explanation involves matters that we have not yet dealt with. At this stage, however, we can say that *atopy is the result of several genes that produce abnormal receptors on the surface of the cells*. This is not a definition you will find in any large medical textbooks in print at the time of writing this book. The knowledge on which it is based is too new to have reached the major texts. So far, it has appeared only in scientific papers and a few medical journals. What does it mean?

Cell receptors are among the most important functional structures of the body and there are hundreds of different kinds. Cell walls are made of aligned fatty molecules such as phospholipids and cholesterol. These stick loosely together like masses of corks floating on a liquid surface. The receptors are much larger protein molecules that are scattered about, lying between the fat molecules and penetrating right through the membrane. Receptors are made in various specific chemical shapes so that the molecules of various substances can latch on to them in the way a piece of a jigsaw puzzle fits into place. Cells have receptors for large numbers of hormones and other substances that can control some function within the cells. Adrenaline, thyroid hormone, insulin and many other substances cause changes to occur in cells by latching on to specific receptors. Most drugs also work by having molecules of just the right shape to latch on to particular receptors.

Some receptors have a different function – to provide a site to which particular antibodies can attach. It is this type of receptor with which we are concerned here. Shortly we shall take a brief look at antibodies and see why they are important in eczema. But, for now, let's concentrate on the abnormal receptors in atopy. When scientists were investigating the genetic basis of atopy, they had no idea that it had anything to do with cell receptors. The work that led to this breakthrough was done in Oxford by a team of British and Japanese

17

scientists led by Julian Hopkins of the Churchill Hospital. This research started in 1985 with a study of the genetics of asthma by examining DNA samples from 100 families with atopy.

By 1989 these scientists had proved that there was a gene or genes for atopy. At least one of these genes was situated on chromosome number 11. After many months of meticulous work they were able, by August 1991, to identify the particular section of chromosome 11 that was implicated. Genes are simply lengths of DNA that instruct cells how to put protein molecules together. Proteins are long strings of small and quite simple molecules called amino acids joined, end to end, in a particular order. Every cell has a good supply of amino acids dissolved in its fluids and the genetic code – the sequence of bases on DNA taken three at a time – indicates which amino acids are to be selected and in what order. There are 20 different amino acids, some or all of which may be used to form a particular protein. Proteins often have thousands of amino acids and all of these must be properly selected and in the right order in the chain. Since our bodies are mostly made of protein, this remarkable process is obviously fundamental to body structure. A great many diseases are caused by a change (mutation) in a normal gene that results in the protein formed being slightly abnormal, and mutant genes are often only very slightly different from normal genes, as we shall see.

The gene variant that causes the abnormal cell receptor in atopy is very common. But, of course we knew that already because we know that millions of people have eczema, asthma and hay fever. What we now know is that a high proportion of people who carry this particular abnormal gene have some kind of symptoms – wheezing, sneezing and watery eyes or itchy, red scaly patches on their skin. At the time of writing, only one abnormal gene has been identified on chromosome 11 and, oddly enough, the inheritance of this gene occurs only through the female line. This presents a problem because we already know that atopy can, although less commonly, be inherited from the father. The researchers, however, are fairly certain that the gene they have isolated is responsible for only some of the cases of atopy, estimated at about 60 per cent. It must be presumed that there is at least one other gene for paternally-transmitted atopy. The experts suggest that half a dozen different genes may be involved in the production of atopy.

The abnormal gene on chromosome 11 is actually responsible for producing an abnormal receptor on the surface of particular kinds of cell found in large numbers in people with eczema, asthma and hay fever. These are the mast cells and the eosinophil cells found in profusion in the deeper layer of the skin, in the air tubes of the lungs and in the lining of the nose and eyes. In people with eczema, there is also considerable current specific interest in the abnormal receptors on the Langerhans cells in the epidermis of the skin. If you have forgotten what these are, turn back to the section on the structure of the skin in chapter 2.

The abnormal receptors on Langerhans cells are not produced by the gene that has been discovered on chromosome 11. But the scientists are pretty sure that other genes are involved in atopy and it is likely that the gene for the Langerhans receptor will be found soon.

What is the change in the receptor?

Most genetic mutations result in the production of a protein that doesn't act properly. Since most of the 100,000 or so proteins produced by the DNA code are enzymes – vital substances which are essential in promoting the thousands of biochemical reactions that keep the body working properly – you can see how readily mutations cause diseases. In the case of the antibody receptor on the mast, eosinophil and Langerhans cells, however, the problem is that it acts all too well. The abnormal receptor is, in fact, far too good at latching on to the antibody concerned, so the particular antibody that is featured in atopic conditions gets stuck on to the mast, eosinophil and Langerhans cells in excessive quantities.

Surprisingly, the mutated gene for the over-enthusiastic cell receptors is only very slightly different from the normal and the protein receptor it produces differs from the normal receptor by only one amino acid. The properties of proteins are critically dependent on the right amino acids being present in the right order. So, although this difference is tiny, it is enough to make the receptor far more sensitive than usual.

19

Why are antibodies relevant in eczema?

Atopy, by itself, is not enough to cause eczema. It merely causes a strong tendency to eczema, asthma, hay fever and some forms of food allergy. The particular way in which atopy reveals itself – eczema, asthma or whatever – tends to run true to type in any particular atopic family. Some families are mainly eczema families; others go in for asthma; others hay fever. Why this should be so remains unexplained in detail, but it seems very likely that particular environmental factors, experienced in common by all members of the family, determine which way things will go.

One of the commonest ways in which the environment attacks the body is, of course, by invading it with germs and other foreign substances. Although knowledge of the environmental factors in eczema is scanty, we know a great deal about them in the other atopic conditions. Foreign substances such as airborne pollens, house dust mite excreta, industrial chemicals and many others are well established factors in the production of asthma and hay fever. You can read all about these in the two Sheldon Press books that are really companion volumes to this book – *Living with Asthma* and *Coping Successfully with Hay Fever*.

The system of the body that protects it from germs and other foreign invaders is called the immune system. This system works by manufacturing antibodies – also known as immunoglobulins. These globulins are soluble proteins which latch on to the invaders, mark them and immobilize them so that the eating and scavenging cells of the system (the phagocytes) can destroy them. The immune system cannot tell whether any tiny item of foreign material is dangerous to the body or not. It just knows that it is different from its own substances (foreign). Every one of our own body cells carries identifying markers – small chemical groups on its surface – which tell the immune system cells that it is 'self' and should be left alone. But when foreign cells or large chemical groups get into the body their identifying flags are missing or different and the immune system immediately attacks them.

Of course, there is nothing conscious about this. The action of the immune system is so remarkable that is is often described in almost human terms of armies and battles. The processes, however, although highly complex, are all automatic and work by virtue of simple chemical linkages (like jigsaw pieces fitting) which cause cells to behave in predictable ways. Free-moving cells of the immune system are chemically attracted to the site of trouble by chemical messengers carried by the blood stream or diffusing in the tissue fluids.

Antibodies are made by a class of cells known as B lymphocytes – B cells for short – and they do an excellent job of protection. There are thousands of different kinds of antibodies, each one exactly right (specific) to tackle a particular foreign invader. They fall into five large groups, or classes, of antibodies designated by various letters. The best known of these groups is group G – the gamma globulins. This contains the main class of antibodies against infection, and that is why gamma globulin is so often used to treat or prevent particular infections. 'Antibody class G' or 'immunoglobulin class G' are rather awkward mouthfuls, so doctors abbreviate the antibody classes to Ig, which stands for immunoglobulin. Gamma globulin can be abbreviated to IgG.

The class of antibodies with which we are concerned when considering atopy is not, however, one of the classes concerned with infection. No one has ever suggested that eczema is an infection any more than asthma or hay fever is. Here we are concerned with the immunoglobulin produced as a result of substances to which we are allergic. These are called allergens. And the class of immunoglobulins involved is class E. For the purposes of this book, we can forget about all the other classes and concentrate on this one, known by all doctors as IgE. IgE, which was discovered in the 1960s, is the allergy antibody class, and most people with eczema or other atopic disorders have far more IgE in their bodies than other people. The normal levels of this protein in the blood are in the region of 250 nanograms per millilitre of blood (a nanogram is one thousand-millionth of a gram). People with hay fever and asthma have up to 2,500 nanograms per millilitre; but people with eczema have up to 25,000 nanograms in each millilitre of blood.

It is the high-affinity IgE receptors that the atopy genes' code produces. We will come shortly to the way in which IgE causes the symptoms of eczema, asthma and hay fever. At this stage it is sufficient to say that, for most of us, IgE seems to be unqualified bad

21

news, and the more we have of it the worse it is for us. From our point of view, everything it does appears to be harmful.

Can IgE do any good?

So what is IgE for? Why should the immune system produce a class of antibodies that seem to serve no useful purpose and only do harm? Well, to answer this question we must first appreciate that the body, as it evolved over millions of years, would not develop a system as complicated as the IgE production system for no reason. Secondly, we must bear in mind that the IgE system is very old. It evolved a very long time ago when life was very different from what it is today.

The best explanation currently available seems to be that the IgE antibody system evolved to cope with parasitic worms. In primitive conditions, all mammals are heavily infested with worms. People with worm parasites have high levels of IgE, so high indeed that there may not be enough left over to cause other IgE effects such as eczema. Populations with a high incidence of worm parasites have a low incidence of atopic disorders such as eczema. This interesting fact was brought out in a paper in the *Lancet*, published as long ago as 1976 by a scientist called J. A. Turton, and entitled *IgE, parasites and allergy*. With recent advances in knowledge, this idea has attracted more attention. There are other scientific reasons to link IgE to worms. Happily, no one has yet, so far as I know, proposed worms as a treatment for eczema, asthma or hay fever.

The system no doubt served an excellent purpose in keeping down parasitization in cave persons, but, unfortunately, we are stuck with it today. IgE is also produced in large quantities in response to a wide range of other unwanted substances such as tree and grass pollens, fungal spores, house dust mite droppings and so on. To explain how IgE does its damage it is necessary to tell you about the mast cells, the eosinophils and the Langerhans cells.

The mast cells and their friends

It seems likely that the mast and eosinophil cell systems evolved as part of the anti-worm campaign. One of the most striking changes that occur in the blood in people with worms is a very large increase in the proportion of eosinophils among the white cells. This is called an eosinophilia and it is so characteristic of worms – as well as of various allergic conditions – that when it is found, one or other of these conditions is immediately suspected. For the purposes of this book we can safely class mast cells and eosinophils together. Incidentally, eosinophils are given this rather bizarre name simply because they so readily take up the red dye eosin. *Phil-* is just the Greek root meaning 'loving', as in 'philanthropist' or 'philanderer'. When eosinophils are stained they assume a striking appearance of bright red spots. These spots are granules, and the mast cells, too, show this feature.

The mast cells were first spotted by the celebrated German bacteriologist Paul Ehrlich (1854–1915) who observed that when they were stained for easy examination under the microscope they were seen to contain lots of small granules that stained densely. Ehrlich thought the granules were material that the cells had eaten and since *Mast* is German for 'animal feed', that is what he called them. Mast cells and eosinophils occur in large numbers all over the body. They are especially prevalent in the skin of eczema sufferers and in the air tubes of people with asthma. They also occur in the noses of people with hay fever.

Chemical microanalysis shows that the granules, from both types of cell, consist of a cocktail of powerful and unpleasant substances most of which cause severe inflammation when they come in contact with other body cells. These substances include histamine, leukotrienes and prostaglandins, all of which are well-known body irritants. Histamine and the leukotrienes are powerful trigger substances that tighten small involuntary muscles. Prostaglandins are released from any kind of cell that is injured, and are the cause of the associated pain. They are used as drugs to cause abortion. The granule contents can be severely damaging to the skin.

The best place for these granules is safely within the cells when they are made. Nature, however, has other ideas. As we have seen, these cells have receptor sites on their surface that fit IgE with particular ease. As a result, when the immune system makes IgE proteins, which it can do at a rate of about 2,000 a second, these molecules soon find themselves firmly latched onto the mast cells and eosinophils. Like all other antibodies, IgE is specially selected to deal with a particular foreign substance and will always, if it can, attach itself to that substance. Let us assume that, in this case, the substance is something from the environment that has managed to get into the body. Unfortunately there is a gap in the story at this point. We do not yet know, for certain, whether there is one particular obscure allergen that causes ordinary infant eczema. There is, however, plenty of evidence that a wide range of substances can act as allergens to produce eczema in different people. We will assume a single allergen and call it substance X.

Whatever substance X may be, the person with atopic eczema has acquired a sensitivity to it. This means that the IgE that is attached to the mast cells is expressly designed to attach also to molecules of this substance. The next time a few particles of substance X come along they will latch on, in no time, to the IgE that is already fixed to the mast and eosinophil cells. Whenever a molecule of this substance links to two adjacent IgE antibodies a strain is applied to the mast cell membrane and it tears open, releasing the granules. Doctors use the impressive term degranulation to describe this process but all it means is that the cell membrane leaks granules. Histamine, leukotrienes, prostaglandins and other unpleasant substances are let out.

These substances released into the skin cause the itching, inflammation and general skin damage that we call eczema. Itching is a major feature and, inevitably, this leads to scratching and further damage to the skin. One of the effects of skin inflammation is the release of watery fluid into the substance of the skin from the blood. This fluid is released in tiny droplets so that the skin cells become slightly separated. The skin is then said to be spongiform and oedematous. This fluid can make its way outwards in a process called exudation until it appears on the surface as blisters of variable size. In atopic eczema these blisters are often small enough to be called vesicles and these are a highly characteristic feature of the eczematous rash. Exudation is not, of course, confined to eczema; it is a feature of other skin disorders and is probably most familiar in the blisters that form after burns to the skin.

What about the Langerhans cells?

We know that in eczema the abnormally 'sticky' IgE receptors occur plentifully on the membranes of the Langerhans cells just as they do on the granular cells. In fact, the Langerhans cells are the only cells in the outer layer of the skin (the epidermis) to carry these receptors. But the Langerhans cells do not act in the same way as mast cells and eosinophils. Degranulation is not their scene. Langerhans cells are what is known as antigen presenting cells. This is a remarkable process. Once the particles are hooked on to the receptors on the Langerhans cells, these cells carry these particles to lymph nodes (commonly known as 'glands'). There they present them to the cells, the lymphocytes, that actually produce the IgE. Obviously, the possession of highly efficient IgE receptors, to which antigen readily attaches itself, greatly helps the Langerhans cells in this process. Langerhans cells are notable for their octopus-like shape. Electron microscope pictures of Langerhans cells show numerous bead-like lumps on the 'tentacles' of the octopus. These are antigen-antibody complexes – combinations of IgE and the particular allergen that causes the eczema.

It requires only a tiny quantity of the allergen to be presented to the lymphocytes by the Langerhans cells to start off this process. Once under way it rapidly leads to an increase in the amount of IgE present. The role of the Langerhans cells has been mainly investigated in connection with contact allergy in adults – a form of eczema dealt with in chapter 5. Because the Langerhans cells are situated in the epidermis they are accessible by allergens, such as tiny particles of nickel, acrylates and poison ivy that can pass into the surface layer of the skin. These substances, by themselves, are not normally allergenic, but as they pass through the skin they become linked to normal body proteins to form a conjugate that can act as a powerful allergen. This is carried by the Langerhans cells to the lymph nodes draining the skin for presentation to the lymphocytes.

More about allergic eczema

There are still many unanswered questions about allergic eczema and especially about the infantile form. Why, for instance, is allergic eczema becoming more common? Why is it increasing at a rate far faster than can be accounted for by an increase in genetic atopy? Why does it nearly always affect the flexures of the limbs – the bends of the elbows and the backs of the knees? No one has the least idea. Again, why is it that the clinical course of eczema is so unpredictable? Why does it quite often disappear altogether in childhood or, in other cases, recur without warning throughout life?

Obviously, there has been considerable interest, in dermatological circles, in the attempt to discover the allergens responsible for infantile eczema. Many people are convinced that they know what precipitates attacks of eczema. Some parents are in no doubt that their child's eczema is brought on by exposure to domestic animals; others are equally convinced that the precipitating factor is the taking of certain foods. Although food allergy is much less common than many popular medical books would have us believe, the possibility that this is a factor in eczema has been investigated, with interesting results.

One recent, carefully conducted trial of possible food hypersensitivity involved what is known as a double-blind, placebo-controlled study. This means that neither the patients nor the people doing the trial know, until afterwards, which of the capsules taken contained the substance thought to cause the trouble and which contained an inert dummy substance (placebo). Thirty-three children with atopic eczema thought to be related to food were tested in trial. When they ate an extract of the food believed to be the precipitating factor, 31 of them (89 per cent) developed itching and diffuse skin eruptions. In 19 of the children there were also other allergic effects such as tummy upsets and wheezing. The symptoms came on between 10 and 90 minutes after the food was taken. Fortunately, there were no alarming or dangerous reactions. The foods causing the reactions in most cases were eggs, milk and peanuts. But the range of possible food allergens was wide, and some children reacted to fish, beef, wheat, rye bread and peas. Other studies have shown that seafood and nuts are also common antigens.

One of the most interesting findings in this trial was that all the children who reacted to food had a significant rise in the level of histamine in their blood. This histamine had to come from mast cells and eosinophils that had been ruptured and degranulated by the combined effect of IgE and the attached food molecules. A rise in histamine in the blood implies an even greater rise in the vicinity of the degranulated mast cells and eosinophils in the skin. No one should be surprised if these children developed itching and local skin inflammation. These children were unusual in the sense that they were already suspected of having food allergy. So the trial told us nothing about how often food allergy is a cause of atopic eczema. There is more about this later in the book.

What else do we know for certain about allergic eczema? Well, we know that it features a number of characteristic abnormalities. These include:

- very dry skin;
- excessive production of keratin scales (see chapter 2);
- lowered threshold to any stimulus that causes itching;
- a strong tendency to produce lichenification (see above) in response to scratching;
- abnormal sensitivity to hormones and drugs that narrow blood vessels;
- reduced ability of the skin to hold water;
- a tendency for the skin to become infected with germs, especially staphylococci.

Staphylococci are the germs that cause boils and abscesses. As we shall see, secondary infection of eczema by staphylococci and other organisms such as herpes simplex virus can be a very serious matter (see chapter 6).

Allergen triggers off eczema

Eczema can be triggered by many different stimuli (allergens). People whose eczema is brought on in this way usually have one particular trigger, or sometimes more than one, and it is especially important to identify these so that they can be avoided, if possible. It can be helpful to have a list of substances that have been proved in the past to act as triggers for eczema. Here is such a list. It is not, of course, comprehensive, but includes most of the best-known allergen eczema triggers.

Naturally occurring triggers

- house dust mite droppings
- tree or grass pollens
- ragweed pollen (especially in the USA)
- fungal spores
- animal hair particle proteins
- animal skin flakes (dander)
- animal saliva
- dried animal urine
- kapok and feather stuffing for pillows, etc.

Manmade triggers

- biological (enzyme-containing) washing powders
- detergents
- fabric softeners
- irritating skin ointments and lotions
- antihistamine creams
- anaesthetic skin ointments or creams
- perfumed skin creams
- creams containing Parabens
- resorcinol ointments or creams
- a few food additives such as tartrazine
- various drugs, especially beta-blockers and aspirin.

Food triggers

- nuts
- shellfish
- some fruits
- yellow split peas
- egg protein
- cow's milk
- wheat
- peanuts
- codfish
- rice
- pork
- betel-nut chewing.

All these can act as allergens promoting the production of IgE and an increase in mast cells and eosinophils in the skin. Probably the most generally important allergic trigger is the house dust mite. Here the actual allergen is a digestive enzyme that coats the mite's dropping. House mite droppings readily become airborne when bedding is shaken or carpets vacuum cleaned. Even if the droppings are introduced into the body by inhalation they can still provoke the skin reaction of atopic eczema.

It may take a bit of detective work to establish a clear association between house dust mite droppings and eczema. Improvement in the eczema after a change of address, a holiday at a different location, or even a spell in hospital, could imply that mites are relevant. These mites cannot survive at altitudes above about 1,000 metres. So if a person's atopic eczema were to clear on an Alpine holiday, for instance, this would suggest that mites were an important factor.

Remember that there are other triggers of eczema besides allergens. These are covered in chapter 10.

A recapitulation

I expect you might well have found this chapter quite hard going. So here is a short recap just to get the main points of the argument in order.

- There is at least one gene on chromosome 11, probably more, which results in abnormal antibody receptors forming on certain cells;
- Some of the cells concerned are called mast cells and eosinophils and these contain granules of very irritating chemicals;
- People with these abnormal receptors on their cells are said to have inherited the condition of atopy;
- Atopic people are prone to develop eczema, asthma or hay fever, or some combination of these;
- Such people have a higher than normal quantity of a particular class of antibodies called immunoglobulin class E (IgE);
- Those with atopic eczema have the highest IgE levels of all;
- IgE attaches unusually easily to the abnormal receptors;

29

- The substances that cause eczema and the other atopic conditions (allergens) become attached to the IgE molecules because the latter are selected by the immune system to fit accurately to the allergens;
- When this happens, the cell membranes are torn and the irritating substances are released;
- If this happens in the skin, the result is the severe itching and skin damage we call eczema;
- There are certain many-tailed cells in the outer layer of the skin called Langerhans cells. These attract the particular allergens causing the eczema and carry them to lymph nodes where there are masses of the cells (lymphocytes) that select and manufacture antibodies. As a result of this presentation of antigens, more IgE is produced;
- There is still uncertainty as to the allergens that cause infantile eczema;
- There is, however, good evidence that, at least in some cases, the allergen is acquired in food that is eaten.

4

The Features of Atopic Eczema

Atopic dermatitis tends to vary in severity from time to time, and in most cases will gradually improve, with or without treatment, with increasing age. A great many children who suffer from it in infancy and early childhood are completely free of symptoms and signs by the time they start primary school.

The condition can conveniently be looked at as it affects people of three different age groups. In some cases, these can also be considered as stages of the disease.

Infancy

Atopic eczema is rare before the age of two months. It may or may not be a coincidence that prior to two months of age the development of the nervous system in babies has not reached the stage at which they have the necessary physical coordination that allows them to scratch.

When it first appears, atopic eczema usually affects the cheeks, forehead and scalp and is distressingly conspicuous. It then tends to spread to the limbs, especially to the wrists and hands. Fortunately, in most cases the rash soon clears from the face and is concentrated on the limbs, although it often persists behind the ears. Most affected toddlers have eczema rash at the bends of the elbows and knees, and many also have a rash on the ankles and the backs of their feet. There is also a tendency for the rash to appear on areas subjected to pressure (such as that caused by sandal straps).

In this age group eczema characteristically features much inflammation, with oozing and crusting. The early months are the worst and the tendency is for the condition to become less severe by the age of two.

Childhood

In some cases, the childhood stage is simply a continuation of the earlier stage. In the others, atopic eczema starts for the first time after the toddler stage. The features of the childhood stage are somewhat different from those of infancy. Instead of the oozing and crusting, the rash is usually drier and marked by the red and white scaly pattern of lichenification (see chapter 1) with obvious scratch-marks. In most cases the affected areas are limited to the bends of the elbows and knees, but in severe cases extensive areas of the limbs are affected and the rash may also appear on the trunk and face.

Another feature of the childhood stage is a characteristic change affecting the mouths of the hair follicles. These become prominent and hardened with tiny 'volcanoes' of heaped-up keratin (see chapter 2). This condition is called keratosis pilaris which just means 'a horny change in the hair situation'. It is easily felt by running the hand over the affected skin, especially on the upper arms.

In the majority of children with atopic eczema the condition clears up spontaneously some time between the ages of two and five. In those in whom it persists, there is commonly a marked improvement around puberty.

Adulthood

Adult atopic eczema tends to become less severe as time passes so that it is rare for people after middle age to be badly affected. The condition can, however, persist even into the 60s. In the majority of cases of adult eczema it is less obviously active than the eczema of infancy. It is a chronic condition characterized by very marked lichenification (see chapter 1) especially at the bend of the elbow and behind the knees. These areas are often excoriated by scratching. Another common site for adult atopic eczema is the nape of the neck. Much less often, eczema may affect the face, hands and the genital region. Tiny, solid skin elevations known as papules (see below) are a common feature of adult eczema and these commonly run together to form larger areas in the characteristic sites.

A number of other features occur. There is a definite increase in the tendency to hives or nettle-rash (urticaria). Affected women commonly suffer dermatitis of the nipples. In adult atopic eczema the creases under the lower eyelids may become more prominent, causing a kind of double pleat that can make the affected person appear tired or even prematurely aged. There is often undue thinning of the outer halves of the eyebrows. Sometimes the palms of the hands have more than the usual number of creases.

The symptoms and signs of atopic eczema

First an explanation of the difference between symptoms and signs. Most people outside the medical profession are unaware that there is such a difference.

A symptom is something experienced only by the individual. One may suspect from a person's expression that he or she is having a symptom, but one cannot be sure that this is actually happening. It is only the sufferer that experiences it. A symptom is purely *subjective*. A sign, on the other hand, is something that another person can actually experience, usually by seeing. A sign is *objective*.

The table below illustrates this. A selection of symptoms is given, and each one is paired with a sign that could be associated with it.

Symptoms	**Signs**
pain	skin rash
itching	scratching
anxiety	breast lump
dizziness	staggering
loss of appetite	loss of weight
nausea	vomiting
depression	expression of sadness

In atopic eczema, the principal symptom is itching. This is so characteristic and important that few doctors would make the diagnosis in the absence of itching. There is, of course, also a range of signs.

Itching

Many sufferers from eczema would be willing to tolerate it were they relieved of the dreadful itching that is such a constant feature of the condition. Itching is the one oustanding symptom of atopic eczema. The itching is not necessarily confined to the areas of the rash but may be generalized. It is, however, mainly localized to the fronts of the arms and the backs of the legs. The severity of the itching varies with the seasons and is often worse in winter. It also varies with the time of the day, being worst in the evenings and least around midday.

Itching is a strange symptom, closely tied up with the state of mind of the person concerned and capable of influencing the state of mind. It may be that the evening increase in itching is more apparent than real and is caused by the relative lack of concentration on important matters connected with daytime work. There is, however, an increased skin blood flow during the evenings and a slight rise in body temperature, and this may be a factor.

It is a common observation and experience that itching can be provoked, or aggravated, by emotional upset or stress. This idea has also been supported by formal research.

The rash

Throughout this book, you will find repeated references to the signs of the various forms of eczema. You will, however, find it convenient, for quick reference, to have a short recapitulation of these in this chapter. There are also some details of the rash which are not dealt with elsewhere in the book.

Papules are tiny dome-shaped elevations in the skin, some 0.5 to 1.5 millimetres in diameter, often with hard keratin points that can easily be felt. They are very variable in number and size but are a common feature of atopic eczema. When especially large and hardened on their points, papules are known as keratosis pilaris. This is especially common on the upper arm and on the sides of the trunk. Papules are commonly associated with dryness of the skin and a general increase in the amount of hardening of the outer layer (keratinization of the epidermis – see chapter 1). This state of excessive thickening of the outer horny skin layer (hyperkeratinization) is known to lower the threshold for itching.

As we have seen, the typical active eczematous rash occurs mainly in infants and children. This features red patches with tiny blisters (vesicles), weeping, crusting and scaling. The edges of these inflamed patches are not distinct, but merge imperceptibly into apparently unaffected skin. Microscopic examination of affected skin patches shows that the cells of the skin are separated by an unusual amount of fluid so that the tissue has become rather spongy. This is called intercellular oedema.

Because of the torturing itch, constant rubbing and scratching is inevitable. The skin responds to this trauma by producing a thicker

34

protective layer of keratin (see chapter 1). This, in turn, becomes excoriated by scratching, producing the appearance known as lichenification. The thickening of the skin makes the normal skin furrows more prominent. Wherever there is scratching, lichenification is liable to occur; and if the scratching becomes widespread, so will the lichenification.

Whitening on pressure

People with atopic dermatitis have an excessive tendency for the small blood vessels of the skin to close down when local pressure is applied to the skin. This strange characteristic can be demonstrated in about 70 per cent of people with atopic eczema by stroking the skin with a blunt-pointed object such as the tip of a Yale key. It is actually possible to produce white writing on the skin of such people. This phenomenon is called white dermographism – a term that simply means 'white writing on the skin'. It indicates that the blood vessels that have been compressed have remained for a time markedly narrowed so that the normal pink appearance of the skin is lost. White dermographism occurs even in areas of the skin that are not affected by eczema.

5

The Other Forms of Eczema

A further note about medical terms is needed at this point. Unfortunately, different doctors sometimes mean different things when they use the terms 'eczema' and 'dermatitis'. In fact, as we have seen, there is no real difference between the two terms, and most dermatologists use them interchangeably. In general, American dermatologists seem to prefer the term 'atopic dermatitis' while British doctors prefer 'atopic eczema'. They are all, however, talking about the same conditions. The 1995 edition of the excellent *Scientific American Medicine* on CD-ROM has a major section headed 'Atopic Dermatitis and Other Eczematous Disorders'.

This chapter is concerned with the forms of eczema or dermatitis that characteristically affect adults and have not been a problem from childhood. They are essentially forms of eczema that result from contact between the skin and any one of a large range of materials acting as allergens. These condition are classified as cases of contact dermatitis.

As we have seen, a proportion of cases of childhood eczema do persist into adult life. These cases have all the characteristics of atopic eczema and these are covered in chapters 1 and 3. But childhood atopic eczema can affect adults even if the disorder does not persist. Here is a case history that illustrates this point.

CASE HISTORY
Abbie's childhood rashes were assumed to be no more than episodes of 'dry skin'. Later events were to show that they had a different and more important significance.

PERSONAL DETAILS
Name Abbie Rubens
Age 27
Occupation Freelance copy-editor
Family Parents alive and well.

MEDICAL BACKGROUND
Abbie has been generally healthy since the age of about five. Prior to that, however, she caused her parents some anxiety because of repeated episodes of cough with marked wheezing. This was diagnosed as bronchitis and was treated with simple cough mixtures. Happily she seemed to grow out of it and has had very little chest trouble since. The only other problem of any note was a tendency to scaliness of the skin especially around the ankles and elbows. Her mother did not think these worth reporting to the doctor and treated them with moisturizing skin creams.

THE PRESENT COMPLAINT
Abbie attends her doctor complaining of a severe rash affecting both hands. This has occurred several times. Abbie is rather obsessive about cleanliness and is terrified that this is some kind of infection caused by germs. As a result, she has been washing her hands excessively and repeatedly.

The rash, which at first was intermittent, now seems to be persistent.

THE CONSULTATION AND EXAMINATION
The doctor takes a detailed history of Abbie's rash and establishes that the first attack occurred more than a year before. It was mild and soon cleared up. Abbie was not troubled for several months and then had another attack. This, too, settled. The present attack started three or four months before. Each of the attacks has featured tiny blisters and a reddish-brown stained appearance, with pain and itching. This is how the latest attack started but the blisters soon cleared leaving the present state of affairs.

The doctor asks Abbie to undress and checks over the whole of her skin. She notes that the rash is confined exclusively to Abbie's hands. The affected skin is dry and roughened and shows many fissured 'hacks' (skin cracks). She asks Abbie to take off her rings and notes with interest that the skin under the rings is unaffected. There are, however, clear indications of skin damage from scratching, especially at the webs of the fingers.

The doctor says that the rash has all the appearances of a chronic contact dermatitis and that it is probably due to detergents in washing-up liquid or to medicated soaps. Abbie agrees that she has been using a medicated soap but insists that she never used it until after the present attack started. Furthermore, there is no question of allergy to detergents as she is always extremely careful to avoid such contacts and always wears gloves when washing up or handling clothes washing powder.

The doctor is puzzled and refers Abbie to a dermatologist.

THE MANAGEMENT IN HOSPITAL OUT-PATIENTS

The consultant also takes a detailed history but this includes questions about Abbie's childhood illnesses. He is especially interested in her early wheeziness and dry skin. He wonders if Abbie can remember whether, as an infant, she was much troubled by itchiness. This strikes an immediate chord with Abbie who tells him that she spent most of her childhood scratching. The specialist asks her about her parents' health and she tells them that they are generally well but that her mother has a lot of trouble with hay fever.

The specialist then checks over her entire skin and examines her hands carefully. He asks her to confirm the statement in the GP's letter that she has always protected her hands by wearing gloves, and she does so. He then surprises her by asking if he can take a sample of blood, explaining that he has reason to believe that she has a genetic condition known as atopy. A check of the levels of certain antibodies in her blood can help to prove this.

Abbie returns two weeks later and is told that the test does indeed show that she has very high levels of IgE. This is a characteristic of atopy.

THE SPECIALIST'S COMMENTS

The consultant explains that people with a history of atopic eczema are no more likely to develop allergic contact dermatitis than anyone else. Indeed, there is some evidence that they are, on the whole, slightly *less* liable to it. They are, however, more susceptible than non-atopic people to ordinary irritant contact dermatitis and have to be very careful to avoid undue trauma to the

38

skin. Atopic people should, for instance, avoid occupations that involve repeated hand washing, because repeated exposure to soap and water is most undesirable. Abbie wonders whether the GP mentioned her obsessive hand washing in her letter to the dermatologist.

The consultant tells her that it is clear from the history and the result of the IgE test that Abbie is markedly atopic. It is highly probable that her 'bronchitis' was actually a mild atopic asthma – a condition commonly not correctly diagnosed in early childhood. She is perhaps lucky that this cleared up in early childhood; many atopic people remain permanently asthmatic.

The cause of Abbie's hand problem remains obscure. It may be that she has a simple adult atopic eczema, but it would be most unusual for this to be confined to the hands and to appear nowhere else on her body. Another possibility is that she might actually have a contact sensitivity to the rubber gloves she has been wearing. Rubber, or some of the materials used in its processing, is a well-recognized irritant. There are many different substances that can affect the hands, however. He has seen patients who have reacted badly to skin creams, such as lanolin, used to treat dry skin.

He advises her to be very careful with her hands. She is to avoid rubber gloves and to use either vinyl polymer gloves or thin, disposable polythene gloves. She is to wash her hands as little as possible, using plain, unscented and unmedicated soap, and to avoid scratching. He assures her that her condition is not due to dirt or infection.

THE FOLLOW-UP

From that time on Abbie's hand problem starts to improve and within a month her hands are clear. The consultant is unhappy that he has not reached a precise diagnosis and suggests, tentatively, that Abbie might be willing to try the same brand of rubber gloves again to see whether the dermatitis recurs. Abbie thanks him but indicates that she is happy to leave things as they are.

Contact dermatitis

There are two large classes of contact dermatitis – those that are caused by the direct irritant action of external substances, and those that are due to allergy to external substances that come in contact with the skin.

Irritant contact dermatitis

This form of eczema is due to substances that interfere with the normal protective barrier function of the epidermis of the skin (see chapter 2). There are many such substances. Some, like strong alkalis, acids and other corrosive materials are so damaging that they produce their effect on a single contact and at the site of contact. Most people, however, are careful to avoid contact with such obviously damaging substances so the majority of cases of direct irritant contact dermatitis occur after repeated contacts with less damaging substances. In such cases the effect is cumulative and it may take some time before recognizable trouble occurs. Note that this is a simple build-up of damage and should not be confused with the repeated exposures needed to produce allergic reactions (see below).

One of the commonest ways in which skin irritants of this kind cause harm is by their action in removing from the surface of the skin, and then from deeper in the skin, the fatty waterproof sebaceous material (sebum) which keeps the skin waterproof and limits the entry of other damaging substances. Detergents and mild alkalis are as capable of emulsifying human sebum as they are of emulsifying fatty material hardened on to a dinner plate. So repeated exposure even to mild washing-up liquid is capable of degreasing the skin of the hands and removing this protective material. Skin systematically treated in this way may develop a very troublesome chronic eczema. This may become complicated by other factors, such as infection. The complications of eczema are dealt with in chapter 6.

Although irritant contact dermatitis may require treatment along the lines detailed in chapter 8, the right approach to this condition is, of course, to avoid it altogether. This is done by ensuring that there is no possibility of direct contact between the offending substance and the skin. In many cases this will require some form of protective clothing, especially suitable gloves.

Allergic contact dermatitis

Although atopic eczema is essentially an allergic condition, people with atopic eczema are not, as might be expected, more likely to acquire allergic contact dermatitis than anyone else. Research has shown that atopic people are actually slightly *less* liable to allergic contact dermatitis than non-atopic people. This is not to say that they do not frequently develop allergic eczema.

It is a feature of all allergies that the effect they produce never occurs on the first contact. Allergy, as we have seen (chapter 3), requires that antibodies of the immunoglobulin class E (IgE) should be produced. Since the allergic effects are due to the interaction between these immunoglobulins and the substance to which the person is allergic, they can only occur on the second or later contact with that substance. This fact can help to distinguish direct contact effects from allergic effects. It must be acknowledged, however, that the first contact with an allergen may have been quite some time before and is often forgotten about.

Allergic contact eczema is very common and affects up to 2 per cent of the population of the Western world. It is especially common in workers in certain industries. Here is a list of the substances to which industrial workers and others are most commonly found to be allergic:

- balsam of Peru
- benzocaine
- BPF resin
- cobalt chloride
- colophony
- Dowicil 200
- ethylene diamine dihydrochloride
- epoxy resin
- formaldehyde
- kathon
- mercapto substances
- mercaptobenzothiazole
- neomycin
- nickel salts

- paraben substances
- paraphenylene diamine
- potassium dichromate
- PPD black rubber mix
- primin
- quinolones
- thiuram substances
- wood alcohols.

All of these substances are used in a standard set of 20 patch tests for allergy. There are, however, very many more substances to which one can become allergic and many of these can be encountered outside an industrial situation – as can some of those in the above list. It is not widely appreciated, for instance, how common and severe allergy to nickel can be. Fortunately, manufacturers of articles worn in contact with the skin have long been aware of this danger and have, when possible, avoided the use of nickel plating on metal. Even so, people still develop a severe eczematous reaction to such articles as watchstraps, watchbacks, metal jewellery such as bracelets and rings, spectacle frames, nickel-plated bra fastenings, and so on.

Another metal that commonly causes allergy is chromium. The metal, in itself, is less liable to cause trouble than some of its compounds. These are commonly used in the processing of leather, and many people have become allergic to their shoes because of this. In such cases, if leather is to be worn, it may be necessary to have shoes specially made from chrome-free leather.

The signs and symptoms of allergic contact dermatitis are exactly the same as those of any other form of eczema. The affected area, which, at first, is the area of direct contact with the allergen, becomes red and itchy and develops small blisters. The area of affected skin soon extends well beyond the area of actual contact and it is quite common for patches of identical eczema to appear on remote parts of the skin that have not been touched by the allergen. Allergic contact dermatitis gets worse and worse with repeated exposure to the causal allergen. The effect of this is to produce a persistent (chronic) state in which the skin becomes dry, scaly and cracked.

In the domestic situation certain allergens, or vehicles for allergenic substances, are particularly likely to give rise to allergic dermatitis if they remain in contact with the skin. These include:

- soaps
- medicated shampoos
- cosmetics
- hand creams
- hair dyes
- hair tonics
- dyes in clothing and shoes
- skin ointments and creams
- eyedrops
- lanolin
- plants, especially primulas
- metal
- rubber
- jewellery.

As always, prevention is better than cure, so the right way to deal with allergic contact dermatitis is to avoid the contact. This implies knowledge of the allergen and, unfortunately, identification is sometimes difficult, because it is by no means always obvious what is causing the trouble. It is often necessary to do patch testing to identify the culprit. Even this can lead to confusion as a person may be allergic to a number of substances.

Other eczematous disorders

There are numerous causes of skin inflammation that can properly be described as eczematous. It is always important for your doctor to make as exact a diagnosis as possible before proceeding to treatment. Distinguishing between the different causes is known as making a differential diagnosis.

Seborrhoeic dermatitis

This is very common in young babies and may resemble atopic eczema. The main feature – a layer of greasy, yellow scales on the scalp (cradle cap), behind the ears, and on the neck – is not characteristic of atopy. Seborrhoeic dermatitis occurs in the first few months of life and has usually disappeared by the end of the first year. Unlike atopic eczema the condition does not cause much itching. Sometimes the condition features red scaly patches at points of frequent skin contact, such as the elbows and armpits. In these cases, the greasy scales may not occur, but there is never any lichenification (see chapter 1).

Seborrhoeic dermatitis need not cause any particular concern. It never does any real harm and is self-limiting.

Dermatitis from habitual rubbing or scratching

It is easy to set up a vicious cycle by getting into the habit of scratching a particular area of the skin. Anyone who does this persistently will damage the skin in such a way as to produce an itch reaction. Thus, the scratch-itch-scratch-itch cycle is set up. If the cause of the original scratching was some kind of psychological upset, the cycle may be very difficult to break. Skin damage caused in this way is called lichen simplex.

Even so, the solution to this problem is somehow to avoid the scratching. Often the best way to do this is to cover up the affected area completely with some kind of bandage or dressing. The resulting difficulty in scratching will remind the sufferer that scratching is not allowed.

Nummular eczema

The term 'nummular' simply means 'coin-shaped' and derives from the Latin word *nummulus*, meaning 'a small coin'. Nummular eczema, sometimes called discoid dermatitis for the same reason, is an adult disorder featuring coin-shaped patches on the skin that vary in diameter from about 4 to 10 centimetres. These patches are slightly swollen (oedematous), often with small blisters and with a moist surface and a tendency to crusting. They occur mainly on the limbs and especially on the backs of the hands and on both legs. The distribution is often symmetrical. The disc-shaped patches may be itchy to a variable degree but, in contrast to atopic eczema, often

44

cause no itching at all. There is no tendency to lichenification (see chapter 1).

The cause of nummular eczema remains obscure, but a paper in the *British Journal of Dermatology* in 1976 suggested that the condition is probably the result of allergy to bacteria. This is, of course, not the same as a skin infection, such as boils, impetigo or cellulitis. This theory is supported by the fact that treatment with antibiotics is often successful.

Varicose eczema

One of the commonest forms of non-atopic eczema is caused by varicose veins. These widened and distorted veins allow pooling and stagnation of blood, especially in the lower parts of the legs, so that there is an inadequate supply of fresh blood bringing oxygen and nutritional materials to the tissues. As a result, the skin in the area of the affected veins becomes swollen, itchy and discoloured. This is called varicose ezcema. In severe cases the lack of skin nutrition may be so great that the skin breaks down locally to form a varicose ulcer. Varicose eczema most typically affects the skin of the ankle above the bump on the inner side. The skin discolouration is caused by iron from red blood cells released into the skin from the damaged veins.

The essential cause of the problem is lack of support to the surface veins and often resistance to the upward flow of blood from pressure on the veins in the abdomen, as in pregnancy. Much can be done to relieve the situation by providing firm, even pressure on the affected veins with well-designed support hosiery. Surgical removal of the surface veins may, however, be necessary.

Skin-to-skin contact dermatitis

People who are considerably overweight often have areas of overlapping skin in which two skin surfaces remain permanently in contact. This occurs mainly in the armpits, under the breasts, and in the groins. Chafing between these surfaces is called intertrigo and it can give rise to dermatitis especially if there is much sweating. Intertrigo is often complicated by secondary infection, especially with the thrush fungus.

The definitive solution, of course, is to lose weight and this will also confer many other advantages. There is no denying, however, that people with intertrigo necessarily have a major weight problem that is not going to be easily resolved.

6

Complications of Eczema

Uncomplicated eczema can be a major misfortune, but it is never a danger to life. Eczema can, however, develop complications and, in rare cases, some of these can be dangerous or even life-threatening. The most important complication of atopic eczema is secondary infection.

Secondary infection

Healthy skin offers a remarkable degree of resistance to the germs that can cause infection. But skin that has been damaged in any way is much more susceptible. This is partly because breaches of the surface of the skin allow germs access to the deeper layers where they can flourish in a warm, moist environment, and partly because skin damage may involve a reduced efficiency of the local functioning of the immune system. This is called local immunosuppression and it is thought to be one of the reasons why skin affected by eczema is more liable to become infected.

A wide range of germs can affect eczematous skin. These include:

- staphylococci, which cause impetigo or boils;
- herpes simplex viruses, which normally cause cold sores or genital herpes;
- human papillomavirus, which causes warts;
- epidermal fungi, which cause athlete's foot, ringworm and other skin fungal infections;
- molluscum contagiosum viruses, which cause small dimple-centred lumps.

In general, secondary infection of eczematous skin by these organisms is more serious than infection, by the same germs, of healthy skin. The greater protection offered to the germs by the damaged surface means that germs can accumulate in far greater numbers than otherwise. Bacteriological studies show that much larger numbers of germs such as staphylococci are to be found in eczematous patches – even in those not obviously showing infection – than occur in normal skin.

The effect of staphylococcal secondary infection is to superimpose a form of impetigo on the eczema patches. This means increased inflammation and a great deal of oozing of discharge and serum, with crusting. In such cases, the lymph nodes ('glands'), to which the particular area of skin drains, will be enlarged and tender and may even be inflamed. In the case of eczema on the arms or hands, the nodes are in the armpit; when there is eczema on the legs, the nodes are in the groin. There are also lymph nodes behind the knees and around the elbows. Involvement of lymph nodes implies a fairly serious degree of secondary infection. In the days prior to the discovery of antibiotics, people with lymph node inflammation often went on to develop blood poisoning (septicaemia) when the germs got into the bloodstream, and this was commonly fatal.

Kaposi's varicelliform eruption

This condition, also known as eczema herpeticum, is probably the most serious complication of all. It is one that should be familiar to every person with eczema and especially to the parents of children with eczema.

Kaposi's varicelliform eruption is a secondary infection of eczema patches with the herpes simplex virus, or occasionally another virus called the coxsackie virus. Before the eradication of smallpox, the condition was commonly caused by the vaccinia virus deliberately given to protect against smallpox. There is now no reason to vaccinate anyone against smallpox and this should never be done. Previously, eczema was one of the main reasons for avoiding smallpox vaccination.

Kaposi's varicelliform eruption is so called because of its resemblance to chickenpox (varicella), but the condition is very much more serious than any attack of chickenpox. It features high fever, severe illness, and an extensive rash with small skin blisters filled with blood. The rash can readily cover almost the whole of the skin surface. Worst of all, the heavy herpes virus infection can involve the brain and the spinal cord.

Fortunately, since the development of the drug acyclovir

(Zovirax), which can be taken by mouth, doctors have had an effective weapon against this most serious complication of eczema. Even so, the death-rate from severe cases is by no means negligible. The importance of knowing about Kaposi's varicelliform eruption lies in the fact that anyone with a cold sore or other manifest herpes simplex infection must stay away from anyone with eczema. For an adult with a cold sore on the mouth to kiss a child with atopic eczema is indefensible and could be excused only on the grounds of ignorance of the dangers.

Exfoliative dermatitis

Exfoliative means 'shedding leaves' and derives from the Latin word *folium*, meaning 'leaf'. Exfoliative dermatitis is a serious condition in which the whole surface of the skin is shed. Very rarely, in adults, this unpleasant and dangerous complication occurs as a complication of atopic eczema. This is fortunately an exceptional occurrence and the condition is usually a complication of drug treatment of various kinds, or of the skin disorder psoriasis. Only about 4 per cent of cases of exfoliative dermatitis occur as complications of eczema.

If it does happen, however, severe exfoliative dermatitis can offer risk to life because the widespread nature of the disorder leads to dangerous loss of fluid, loss of the ability to control body temperature, and heart failure. It is mentioned here only for completeness and is so rare that it is not a possibility that need cause concern.

Cataracts

A cataract is a loss of transparency of the internal lens of the eye – the tiny, fine-focusing lens that lies behind the pupil. Cataract has nothing to do with the cornea, which is the main outer lens of the eye. There does appear to be a relationship between cataracts and long-standing, widespread atopic eczema; this claim is certainly made in a number of textbooks. Cataracts, which are comparatively rare except in elderly people, seem to develop, on average, five years after the onset of severe eczema. There are conflicting views about how often this happens, and different reports suggest that cataract occurs in anything from 2 per cent to 17 per cent of eczema cases.

However, it is important to appreciate that in people past middle age with a lifelong history of atopic eczema one is not really justified in concluding that cataract development is due to the eczema. The fact is that almost everyone who lives long enough develops some degree of cataract, and most people over 70 have at least a minor degree of visual impairment from cataract. This occurs so gradually that it is seldom noticed until a fairly advanced stage.

The connection between eczema and cataract is said to be supported by the fact that the lenses of the eyes and the skin develop from the same primitive fetal tissue, the ectoderm. But it must be said that many important parts of the body, such as the whole of the nervous system and part of the reproductive system, also develop from the ectoderm. And there is no evidence that eczema arises from some disorder of the ectoderm. The fact that many elderly people with persistent atopic eczema develop cataracts is, in itself, no proof that there is any connection between the two. Many people with warts or skin tattoos also develop cataracts but no one would suggest that these things cause cataracts.

There is, however, one connection between eczema and cataracts that should be noted. The long-term use of steroid drugs, especially if taken by mouth, *can* increase the tendency to cataract formation. Steroids applied to the eyelids or to the skin around the eyes also increase the risk. For this reason, people on intensive treatment for severe atopic eczema should have regular examinations by an ophthalmologist who can check the state of the lenses with a slit-lamp microscope.

7

The Emotional Dimension

Eczema is an emotive subject. Parents are distressed to see the beauty of their young children's skin marred by it and upset by the obvious signs of their discomfort. Sufferers are mentally tormented by itching and embarrassed and mortified by the cosmetic damage. Everyone is troubled by the appearance of a severely affected victim of the disease. But there are other ways in which the emotions are involved.

The skin and the mind

To think of the skin as merely a passive covering for the body is greatly to underestimate its sensitivity to the state of the mind. The skin is, in fact, often an impressionable mirror of the thoughts. The most obvious instance of this is the way in which it reacts to emotions such as embarrassment or fear. Many young people are distressed at their inability to conceal their thoughts because of the way these are revealed by blushing. The cold sweat of terror and even the reflex 'standing up on end' of the body hair under the influence of the arrector pili muscles (see chapter 2), are cases in point.

But the matter is even more subtle than this. The nerve endings in the skin that promote the itch or tickle sensation can be stimulated into producing an itching sensation by purely psychological factors, even in the absence of any external stimulus. It is often a source of amusement to teachers that when biology students are first shown, under the microscope, certain ectoparasite organisms such as mites or body lice, some of them immediately start itching. Similarly, if for any reason you are prevented from scratching, the mere knowledge that this is so is liable to induce itching.

Experiments have repeatedly shown that the severity of the skin changes that occur in acute allergic conditions such as nettle-rash or hives (urticaria) – changes such as the production of purplish weals – can be markedly affected by the state of the mind. Anxiety or tension can make them worse; relaxation and calmness can reduce the severity. The same applies to other skin reactions such as the exudation of fluid (see chapter 3). This is not new knowledge. Indeed

51

the link between mind and skin was so obvious to early dermatologists that they assumed that a number of conditions were primarily caused by mental upset and used terms such as 'angioneurotic oedema' or 'neurodermatitis'. These terms are now deemed old-fashioned and are criticized as seeming to claim too much. But there is still a sound basis of fact behind them even if it remains difficult to quantify or fully explain. In the light of modern advances in immunology it is also no longer considered scientifically respectable to suggest that there is a neurotic basis for certain skin disorders. But every dermatologist will agree that it is only too easy to underestimate the power of the mind on the skin.

The emotional component in itching

Itching is the most important symptom of eczema, and severe itching is a cause of considerable mental distress. At the same time, emotional stress arising from any cause can provoke and aggravate itching and scratching. To a person suffering from eczema, the disease itself may be a profound source of emotional stress. The stage is thus set for the production of a particularly vicious cycle that can be very damaging. Here is a case history that well illustrates this point.

CASE HISTORY
Andrew's eczema had always been of the very mildest until, inexplicably, it started to become severe. The reasons are by no means apparent . . .

PERSONAL DETAILS
Name Andrew Hobbes
Age 22
Occupation Postgraduate philosophy student
Family One brother; parents alive and well.

MEDICAL BACKGROUND
Andrew's health has never caused anxiety. He had the usual childhood infections but soon recovered. The only feature of any note is a very mild eczema affecting the back of his knees and causing little trouble. His parents, too, are generally healthy

although his mother suffers fairly severely from hay fever during the pollen season. His older brother is believed to be well but has lived in India for nearly ten years and little has been heard from him.

THE PRESENT COMPLAINT

During a long vacation from Oxford, Andrew is persuaded by his mother to consult their family doctor as she is sure his eczema has got much worse.

THE CONSULTATION

The doctor, who has hardly seen Andrew before, observes that he is a quiet, reserved, highly intelligent young man who appears to be in good health. He is slightly under-weight but seems active. He is fond of long, solitary walks and gets an adequate amount of exercise in this way, in spite of his studious lifestyle. He is remarkably diffident about his complaint and, in answer to questions, is inclined to dismiss it as unimportant. He seems unusually reluctant to undress when asked to do so.

When the doctor sees Andrew's body he is mildly shocked at the severity and extent of the eczema. Andrew's hands and face are spared but much of the rest of his skin is covered in a markedly lichenified and excoriated rash with patches of blistering here and there. At first the doctor thinks this is a case of ichthyosis but closer inspection shows that it is a simple chronic eczema of the atopic type. The only area that is entirely free is a patch between Andrew's shoulder blades.

The doctor takes a history of the complaint and Andrew admits that he had almost no eczema at all until about a year before. He relates how, during the past year, the rash has gradually but inexorably spread – first to the elbows and arms, then to most of the surface of both limbs and finally extending to the trunk. The last part to be affected has been the skin of the back.

The doctor enquires about itching and at this Andrew smiles wryly and confesses that he had not believed an itch could become such a central part of his life. Controlling the tendency to scratch has become a major preoccupation to be managed only by intense

53

concentration on philosophic problems. Reviewing the distribution of the rash, the doctor notes that the only part of the skin unaffected is the area Andrew cannot easily reach with his fingers.

The doctor now asks Andrew whether anything happened prior to the start of the spread of the rash – anything that might have a bearing on it. Andrew is silent for long time then, with a little encouragement, starts to talk. He explains that, a year ago, he had a letter from his brother who is living as a beggar in Mysore. At the end of the letter, in a postscript, his brother mentioned casually that he had contracted leprosy and was being treated in a Government clinic, but asked him to say nothing about it to their parents. The news greatly distressed Andrew, and on the day he received the letter his skin began to itch. Since then he has found it impossible to avoid scratching. Whenever he has scratched, the rash has appeared and, within a few days, has become established. In this way it has extended all over his body. Andrew seems relieved to be able to talk and finds the doctor's response sympathetic. He has become convinced that he may have been infected from the letter, and asks if the rash is leprosy.

THE DOCTOR'S COMMENTS

The doctor assures him that there is no question of that. In the first place, leprosy affects the body in a totally different way – which he describes – and in the second place, leprosy could not possibly be transmitted by a letter. It takes many years of close physical contact with an affected person to acquire the disease. The doctor goes on to explain that itching is readily provoked by mental stress and that an eczematous rash is readily provoked by scratching. Eczema itself causes severe itching, which provokes scratching. Andrew has become the victim of a common vicious cycle.

The doctor asks Andrew if he would be willing to participate in an experiment. He would like to see whether the rash can be cured without any physical treatment other than that directed to the relief of the itching. He would propose a lubricant bath oil to be used daily, a water-based emulsion to be used instead of soap and a mild antihistamine to be taken at night. The antihistamine will also help to promote sleep. There must, of course, be an absolute veto on scratching and this is to be a point of honour.

Andrew enthusiastically agrees.

THE FOLLOW-UP

Andrew is as good as his word and succeeds, by a strong effort of will, in avoiding scratching. After a few days of heroic effort he is encouraged in this by the observation that the whole rash is becoming definitely less itchy. It takes nearly three months, however, for the rash to disappear, but when it does Andrew's skin is left unblemished. He does not even have the usual patches behind his knees.

Other emotional effects

Many people with atopic eczema and other obvious skin diseases have, whether they acknowledge it or not, a fear of being considered unclean or infectious and thus being socially rejected. This is not surprising. The skin is by far the most conspicuous of all the organs and it is an almost instinctive tendency to react unfavourably, or even aggressively, to perceived abnormality. There are plenty of instances of this throughout the history of the human race. The biblical attitude to leprosy is a case in point.

Such attitudes are, however, largely inappropriate and the result of ignorance. Atopic eczema has nothing to do with lack of cleanliness and it is not, of course, infectious. But these truths are of scant comfort to the sufferer who is well aware of public attitudes and who may even share the popular prejudices and ignorance. Public perceptions of skin diseases such as eczema make it difficult for sufferers to get employment in many occupations. There is no actual medical objection, for instance, to a person with uncomplicated eczema from working as a food handler or in food preparation, but many people are barred from these and other occupations on account of eczema.

Awareness of other people's attitudes can have an extremely depressing effect on the mind and personality of those with eczema. One of the most important things that the friends and associates of eczema sufferers can do to relieve emotional distress is to make no distinction, in terms of touching, between people with eczema and those free from skin trouble. It is very distressing, for instance, to a person with eczema to notice that others avoid shaking hands. And it is often comforting for such people to meet a dermatologist who is obviously completely relaxed about stroking and feeling the skin both in its affected and non-affected areas. Children with eczema commonly suffer as much from social deprivation as from the skin problem. Other children may taunt them and refuse to hold their hands. Between people in a more intimate relationship, this point is of particular importance. Physical contact is a vital part of any such relationship. It is a token of the attitude between people, and if contact is avoided the relationship is liable to be damaged. This applies much more widely in the relationship than just the sex life, of course. It is to be hoped that knowledge of the facts can dispel fear and that books of this kind may do something to help.

Ignorance of the real nature of skin diseases such as eczema is very common among the sufferers themselves. For some reason, there is reluctance to recognize that the skin is an organ and to attribute the disorder to a defect in the skin itself. Conditions like eczema are taken to be due to some other, internal, disorder such as some unspecified toxic effect, an upset of the liver or an impurity in the blood. Errors of this kind simply deprive the affected person of the chance of getting to the root cause of the skin disorder.

8

How Eczema Is Treated

While this chapter contains a good deal of practical and useful information, it is not intended to be a do-it-yourself guide to treating eczema. That is a matter for your doctor. This chapter will certainly help you to achieve the most effective management of the disorder, but its main purpose is to ensure that you are as fully aware as possible of the kinds of treatment available, how they work, and the reasoning behind them. Only if you have this knowledge will you be able to take an informed interest in the treatment prescribed by your doctor.

Regrettably, it has to be admitted that there is no magic cure for eczema. A great deal can be done, however, to keep it under control so that it is reduced to a state of minimal severity. Given proper understanding of the principles of treatment, eczema can almost always be managed successfully. The objectives of treatment are to restore the skin to a normal appearance and function. To achieve this it is necessary to reduce inflammation, to relieve and, if possible, to prevent itching, to reduce the likelihood of complications such as infection and to minimize the particular kind of skin damage known as lichenification.

Although the management of eczema must always be a medical responsibility, it is also a cooperative enterprise in which the affected person or, in the case of a child, the parents must be involved. Research has shown that results are improved if those involved are well informed.

Direct treatment of the skin

Treatment applied directly to the skin is known as topical therapy. The term 'topical' is derived from the Greek word *topos*, meaning 'a place' and appears in words such as 'topography' – the study of the earth's surface features – and 'topology' – the branch of mathematics concerned with surfaces. Topical therapy is by far the most important kind used in eczema and is applied for a variety of reasons. These include:

- suppressing inflammation;
- keeping the skin adequately moisturized (hydrated);
- preventing itching and scratching;
- reducing the number of skin bacteria to minimize the risk of infection;
- removal of discharge and crusts.

In severe cases, all of these requirements may have to be met.

Suppressing skin inflammation

The most powerful and effective anti-inflammatory drugs are the corticosteroids. These have a most important part to play in the management of eczema. The general idea in using steroids is to apply the weakest preparations that will do the job. In addition, use of steroids can be minimized by alternating them with purified coal-tar derivative preparations that also relieve inflammation.

In very severe flare-ups it may be necessary to use quite potent steroids and these will nearly always give prompt relief, so they need seldom be used for longer than a week or so at a time. As soon as a good response has been achieved a milder steroid is substituted for a time and then, when a reasonable clearance of the rash has occurred, steroids are stopped altogether. If new patches of eczema appear, the administration of steroids may have to be resumed intermittently to keep them in check.

Because steroids, especially the more potent ones, do eventually lead to atrophy and thinning of the skin, broken veins, and purplish streaks (striae) similar to those occurring in pregnancy, it is especially important to avoid their use, if possible, on the face. They should also be kept out of skin folds where absorption is greater.

Keeping the skin moist

This is most important and is tackled in two ways. The main cause of loss of fluid from the skin is damage to the epidermis (see chapter 2). Continued application of skin moisturizers and softeners may be necessary to hydrate the skin and to preserve the epidermal barrier that keeps water in. In addition to topical treatment you should remember that, contrary to what you may think, excessive washing makes skin dryness worse, and this increases the tendency to itching. For this reason, the long, luxurious soak in a hot bath or the prolonged session under a hot shower are not to be recommended. Soaps are also liable to remove water from the skin. So try to avoid all unnecessary exposure to water and use a soap substitute, such as cetyl alcohol in a propylene glycol base, for skin cleansing.

There are many different skin moisturizers. Preparations commonly used by dermatologists contain urea (e.g. Aquadrate, Nutraplus), or compounds of urea, glycolic acid, and ammonium lactate. Such preparations also help to smooth the skin and are especially useful in the condition of keratosis pilaris (see chapter 4).

A great many skin moisturizing and anti-itch preparations are available. The wide range is useful as it allows the most suitable, and the least likely to cause skin sensitization, to be selected by experience. They are all available without prescription. In general, creams are water-soluble and ointments are greasy and water-repellent; but this rule is occasionally broken by ointments with a water-miscible base. Ointments may be found more effective than creams if the skin is very dry. The ingredients most commonly occurring in the wide range of over-the-counter products are urea, which attracts and retains water; calamine and zinc oxide, which are soothing to the skin; and weak carbolic acid (phenol), camphor and menthol, which have a mild anti-itch action.

Here is a selection of preparations listed by category:

CREAMS
- Alcoderm cream
- Aquadrate
- Aqueous cream
- Aveeno cream
- Blisteze
- Blistex
- Caladryl cream
- Cepton
- Clearasil
- Conotrane cream
- DDD medicated cream
- Dermacare cream
- Diprobase cream
- E45 cream
- Emulsiderm
- Eskamel cream
- Eurax cream
- Hewletts cream
- Humiderm
- Hydrome Emollient
- Hydromol cream
- Lacticare

- Masse
- R.B.C. cream
- Sudocrem
- Ultrabase cream
- Valderma cream

LOTIONS
- Alcoderm lotion
- Caladryl lotion
- DDD medicated lotion
- Dermacare lotion
- Dermalex
- Eurax lotion
- Keri Therapeutic lotion
- Panoxyl 5 and 10

OINTMENTS
- Calendolon ointment
- Cocois scalp ointment
- Emulsifying ointment
- Kamillosan ointment
- Unguentum Merck

OILS
- Alpha Keri bath oil
- Aveeno bath oil
- Aveeno Oilated
- Balmandol
- Balneum
- Balneum Plus
- E45 Dermatological Bath Oil
- Lipobase
- Morhulin
- Oilatum Emollient
- Oilatum Plus
- Savlon Bath Oil

Preventing itching

The corticosteroids are the most effective drugs here. Topical steroids, even the mildest of them, act like magic in relieving itching. The effect is almost immediate and is so remarkable that there is a risk that steroids will be overused. There are other ways of relieving itching and these should be adopted to the full, while the big guns are kept in reserve. Remember that unduly dry skin promotes itching so every effort should be made, as described above, to keep the skin moist.

Another class of drugs that can be used to prevent itching are some of the tricyclic antidepressant drugs that also act as antihistamines. These are effective in relieving the itching caused by the histamine released from mast cells (see chapter 3). The drug doxepin (Sinequan) used topically in a cream has been shown to be effective in the relief of itching in atopic eczema. Coal-tar preparations can also be used to relieve itching.

Reducing bacteria

The main concern, here, is secondary infection with staphylococci (see chapter 6). It is also important to bear in mind that the extent to which the skin is likely to be contaminated with staphylococci is largely determined by the severity of the eczema. The reasons for this are given in chapter 6. Any measure that reduces this severity – such as the use of topical steroids – will also reduce the probability of secondary infection.

Removing discharge and crusts

This is not very often necessary, but in the acute stage, when there is much exudation (see chapter 3) that dries and crusts over, an effective measure is to apply wet gauze dressings soaked in a solution of aluminium acetate (Burow's solution) and left for ten minutes twice a day. Once the surface is clean a broad-spectrum antibiotic ointment such as mupirocin (Bactroban) is applied to the raw surface.

Light therapy

A proportion of people with atopic eczema discover, usually by chance observation, that sunbathing helps. People who respond in this way can often be improved by a formal course of controlled exposure to ultraviolet light of a suitable wavelength (UVB) to produce tanning. This is called phototherapy. Note that this is not always helpful; indeed some people with atopic eczema actually get worse if exposed to UVB. In those cases, improvement may be achieved with a course of the longer wavelength UVA.

There is a class of drugs known as the psoralens that are used in conjunction with ultraviolet light exposure. This method is known as PUVA (psoralen, ultraviolet A) therapy. Psoralen drugs are plant derivatives such as coumarin or methoxalen which, when applied to the skin or taken internally, increase the tendency of the skin to darken (pigment) under the action of ultraviolet light. This effect can be exploited in the treatment of atopic eczema. Unfortunately, the eczema often recurs after PUVA treatment is stopped. Some dermatologists advise against excessive ultraviolet treatment because of the increased risk of skin cancer. The difficulty here is to decide what is excessive, and the advantages must be balanced against the risks.

Treatment by mouth

Few people suffering from eczema require regular treatment by mouth, but for those unfortunate enough to be very severely affected, oral treatment can be invaluable. Occasional oral treatment to supplement standard topical treatment can also be useful for those less seriously affected.

Antihistamine drugs

Many people with eczema have serious difficulty in breaking the insidious itch-scratch-itch-scratch cycle. For those whose skin state is being made much worse by this process regular use of certain antihistamines can be helpful. Antihistamines used for this purpose may be selected to take advantage of their secondary effect of causing sleepiness. These are especially useful in people who are being kept awake at night by itching. Popular antihistamines for this purpose include hydroxyzine (Atarax, Ucerax) or diphenhydramine (Nytol). Incidentally, diphenhydramine is also often used as a local application for itching. One popular formulation is Caladryl cream or lotion in which the antihistamine is combined with calamine and camphor.

If the anti-itch effect is required without sedation, one of the newer non-sedating antihistamines, such as loratidine (Clarityn) can be used. Different people are best suited by different antihistamines, so a little experimentation may be needed.

Other anti-itch drugs

The opium derivative papaverine, normally used as a muscle relaxant, has a useful effect against itching. It can, when necessary, be taken four times a day and is also formulated, in the USA, as a time-release capsule. Papaverine is not used as a primary treatment for itching, but as a supplement to standard topical treatment.

Steroids

Steroids by mouth or injection (systemic steroids) are *not* used on a long-term basis to treat atopic eczema. In particularly difficult cases of severe and intractable atopic eczema, however, a brief period of treatment with steroids by mouth may be considered. Steroids on the skin are widely accepted as necessary and are considered generally safe because, properly used, absorption into the bloodstream is minimal. Steroids by mouth, unless in very small dosage, inevitably raise the risk of undesirable side effects. There is another reason for this general veto – the probability that when the steroids are stopped the condition may quickly recur as bad as ever, or worse. This is called the rebound phenomenon.

You should know something about the side effects of systemic steroids. If taken in high doses for long periods they will inevitably cause side effects. It would be quite wrong to suggest that all the effects listed below will necessarily occur, but any or all of them are possible. The more important of the side effects include:

- suppression of the body's production of natural steroids
- reactivation of latent infections
- increased susceptibility to new infections
- breakdown of partly-healed stomach or duodenal ulcers
- 'moon face'
- excessive hairiness (hirsutism)
- softening of the bones (osteoporosis)
- diabetes
- high blood pressure
- glaucoma
- cataract.

Suppression of natural steroid production usually occurs if the dose of steroids is equivalent to more than about 7.5 milligrams of prednisolone per day. This causes no harm so long as steroids are being taken, but suddenly stopping the treatment is very dangerous. All patients on long-term systemic steroid treatment should carry a card indicating, in detail, the treatment they are having. In the event of a severe accident or other major stress, this knowledge can be life saving.

The decision to give steroids to young children long-term must be balanced against the fact that these drugs cause severe stunting of growth.

Antibiotics

When eczematous skin is excoriated by scratching it generally becomes infected, usually by staphylococci. This, of course, makes the eczema worse and intensifies the itch. In such cases, antibiotics by mouth may be necessary to control the secondary infection. Indeed, some dermatologists insist that excoriation of the skin is, in itself, an indication that systemic antibiotics are needed.

Before this is done, it is best to culture organisms from the skin so that they can be identified and their susceptibility to selected antibiotics determined. Antibiotics commonly used for this purpose include erythromycin (Erythrocin, Erythromid, Erythroped), cloxa-cillin (Orbenin) and cephalexin (Ceporex, Keflex). Infections that persist in spite of systemic antibiotic treatment suggest that the person concerned might be harbouring resistant staphylococci in his or her nose. This can be established by taking a swab and culturing it. If proved, the infection can be eradicated by a nasal antibiotic ointment or by a special combination of antibiotics by mouth.

Immune system intervention

The most advanced forms of treatment for eczema – many of them still experimental – involve therapies directed at some of the complex immune system processes that underlie the disease (see chapter 3).

One class of substances that seems to promise well is the range of natural hormones known as the interferons. These can now be made by genetic engineering and are becoming much more plentiful. One of the interferons, interferon gamma, acts to prevent the production of the immunoglobulin IgE by B cells (see chapter 3). As we have seen, this immunoglobulin is an essential agent in the degranulation of mast cells and the release of skin-damaging substances in atopic eczema. Research into its use as a treatment for eczema has shown that it can produce a marked clinical improvement. Some of the people treated maintained the improvement for three months after the treatment was stopped. Those taking part in the trial used skin moisturizing medication but no topical steroids. About half the people treated for their eczema in this way had an improvement estimated at 50 per cent. There were, however, some side effects such as muscle aches, headaches, slight fever and some brief reduction in the white blood cell count. Interferon alpha has also shown promise in the treatment of eczema.

One of the most important and widely used immune system controlling drugs is cyclosporin. This powerful drug is routinely used in organ transplantation to prevent graft rejection. Cyclosporin, taken by mouth, has been reported to be highly effective in controlling atopic eczema. Whether one is justified in using such a potentially dangerous drug is, however, another matter entirely. Drugs that interfere so radically with immune system function will always reduce, to some extent, the ability of the person concerned to resist infection. In short, they produce a degree of acquired immune deficiency. Whether cyclosporin, or an associated drug, will become a standard treatment for severe atopic eczema remains to be seen. Much more research is required before drugs of this kind can be regarded as safe for routine use. In the meantime they are best regarded as being appropriate only for exceptionally difficult cases.

General schemes of treatment

Individual doctors, of course, have their own ideas on the details of the treatment of eczema and the management will vary from case to case, depending on the particular features. But there are certain basic principles that apply generally. In all cases it is important for the people concerned or, in the case of children, their parents, to be familiar with all reasonable measures to avoid eczema. These are dealt with in chapter 10.

Mild eczema

In children, a priority is to control itching. This is best achieved by using antihistamines in palatable syrup form. This is given mainly at night, but can be used during the day also, if necessary.

In mild atopic eczema the aims are to avoid infection and control inflammation. These two objectives can usually be achieved by means of an ointment containing a combination of a mild steroid and an antibiotic or antimicrobial agent. If there is no tendency to infection, low-potency steroids may be used alone. The mild steroid hydrocortisone, available in a low-percentage formulation without prescription, is generally safe and is widely used. Hydrocortisone is available in a wide range of preparations, either alone or in combination with antibacterial agents.

Doctors are careful to avoid using powerful steroids, even topically, in young children. These should never be used in mild cases. They are especially careful not to use them on the face or other visible areas as these drugs can quickly cause marked 'broken veins' (telangiectasia) and atrophy of the skin. If mild steroids fail, occlusive dressings with tar or ichthammol (see also below) are used.

Dry skin is consistently treated with an emollient (see above). This can significantly reduce the amount of topical steroids needed.

Treatment of severe eczema

Here is an outline scheme of treatment of the kind adopted by many dermatologists to deal with severe atopic eczema.

Severe cases are best dealt with in hospital. This removes the patient from habitual sources of allergen and allows better facilities for investigation and treatment. Eczematous discharge with crusting is cleared by putting the patient in a tepid bath of water containing bath oil and sometimes wheat bran or colloidal oatmeal (Aveeno). Alternatively, wet gauze dressings, soaked in Burow's solution, can be used, as described above.

While the affected surfaces are being cleared of exudate, an assessment is made of the probability of secondary infection. If there is any indication of this, the infecting agent must be identified and antibiotics or antiviral drugs given. Secondary infection with herpes simplex is treated with acyclovir (Zovirax).

Once the skin is clear of infection, topical steroids are applied. It is bad practice to use steroids in the presence of infection as these encourage its spread. The consensus of opinion is that, in severe cases, powerful steroids – those of high or intermediate potency – should be used at first to produce a rapid resolution of the rash, to restore, as soon as possible, the skin's integrity as a barrier to water and other materials, and to restore its resistance to allergens and irritant substances. These are usually applied twice a day and it is seldom necessary to continue with strong steroids for longer than a week. In many cases, three days of treatment are sufficient. This is important, because the shorter the time, the less likelihood of undesirable side effects. Once a good response is achieved, a less potent steroid can be substituted or the intervals between applications can be lengthened.

Any patches that seem resistant to steroids will usually do better if the ointments are covered with bandages (occlusive dressings). Steroids under bandages are generally more effective than if left exposed. Also, the bandages are helpful in preventing scratching. A determined scratcher will, however, get at the skin whatever is done. The occlusive dressings are often impregnated with zinc oxide and coal tar (Coltapaste, Tarband) or ichthammol (Ichthopaste, Ichtha-band) and can be left in place for as long as a week. Sometimes impregnated bandages are used without steroids, even in quite severe cases, and these may be sufficient. But, as a rule, topical steroids are necessary.

Hints and tips

As we have seen, keeping the skin well moisturized (hydrated) is very important. This does not mean, however, that it is a good idea to sit in a hot bath twice a day. Excessive bathing, especially in very hot water and with lots of soap and foam, will actually *reduce* the hydration of the skin by extracting the natural sebaceous oil (sebum) that keeps the water in. At the same time, undue avoidance of bathing is undesirable as it will increase the probability of secondary infection. So the answer is to bath in moderation, using lukewarm water and minimal soaping and to ensure that, after bathing, you apply oily moisturizing cream to compensate for any loss of sebum.

A pleasantly soothing addition to the bath, which is a safe remedy for the inflammation and a possible substitute for soap, is wheat bran or colloidal oatmeal. Two cupfuls of colloidal oatmeal added to a not too deep bath of lukewarm water has a distinct anti-flammatory, as well as cleansing, effect. Colloidal meal is finely ground and

67

forms a suspension in water. You can put some inside a wash-cloth, dip it in water, squeeze it and use it instead of soap.

Watch out for conditions of excessive atmospheric dryness as these will always increase the rate of water loss from the skin. During cold spells the relative humidity of the air drops. This is because the amount of water vapour in the air rises with a rise in temperature and drops with a fall, as a result of changes in the evaporation rate. The environment that really matters, of course, is that next to the skin. So suitable layered clothing that limits access of outside air can be a great help in the winter time. Cotton underclothes are much to be preferred to wool or synthetics. Wear clothes that tighten at the wrists and neck and use gloves and scarves.

Sudden change of temperature is also undesirable as this frequently triggers itching. This applies both to going outdoors from a warm house and moving from hot to cold rooms indoors. Stepping into a hot bath or shower will also trigger itching. Wrap up well before going out into the cold; wear layered clothing – string vests under less permeable underclothes are useful – and wear a hat or cap.

9

Evening Primrose Oil and Traditional Chinese Remedies

Great public interest has been aroused in the possibility that a harmless oil derived from the seeds of the evening primrose *Oenothera biennis* can help to reduce the severity of atopic eczema. The manufacturers of this product have claimed great things for it. Their promotional literature states that evening primrose oil produces 'a substantial and highly significant clinical improvement' in atopic eczema. There have, however, been conflicting claims for the product, which is expensive and has to be used for long periods, so it is obviously important to know as much as possible about it. Eczema is not the only condition for which this oil is recommended. It has been promoted for the treatment of premenstrual tension, menopausal flushing, Raynaud's phenomenon, painful breasts, rheumatoid arthritis, multiple sclerosis, hyperactivity, schizophrenia and other conditions. Doctors are always suspicious of universal panaceas and there are conflicting opinions on the value of evening primrose oil in these conditions also.

Evening primrose oil

To form a reasonable judgement on whether evening primrose oil is likely to be useful in eczema, you will first need a bit of background information.

The significance of fats in the skin

People with atopic eczema usually have dry skin that is not as good as it should be at keeping water in. This is part of the reason for the dryness. They also show, as we have seen, small, horny bumps around the hair follicles, like hardened goose pimples – the condition called keratosis pilaris – and a general tendency to scaliness known as ichthyosis (*ichthos* is Greek for 'fish'). Unfortunately, eczema causes such itching that affected people almost always scratch a lot and this causes further scaliness. So it is sometimes difficult to distinguish primary from secondary effects.

There is clear evidence, however, that much of the flakiness and dryness of the skin in atopic eczema is due to changes in the oil content of the skin. Research has shown that eczema involes definite abnormalities in fat processing in the skin. It has been known for a long time that fats are necessary for healthy skin. As long as the late 1920s it had been shown that rats fed on a completely fat-free diet developed redness, scaling and itching of the skin, just like eczema. Later it was found that human patients who were having to be fed directly into the bloodstream (parenteral feeding) developed similar changes if the feed did not contain essential fatty acids.

Fat molecules consist of a 'backbone' of glycerol (glycerine) to which is attached three fatty acids. For this reason fats are called triglycerides. Different fats differ by reason of the different kinds of fatty acids that are attached to the glycerol backbone. Incidentally, when we talk about saturated and unsaturated fats – a matter of single or double bonds between adjacent carbon atoms – it is really the fatty acids that are either saturated or unsaturated. Here we are concerned with the actual *kinds* of fatty acids. There are many of these, but the two fatty acids that are essential for keeping people and animals alive and healthy are called linoleic acid and alpha-linolenic acid. Trials showed that it was deficiency of these unsaturated fatty acids that was responsible for the skin changes. Patients with these eczema-like skin effects could be put right simply by rubbing some linoleic acid into the skin.

Essential fatty acids and eczema

Since the skin changes caused by fatty acid deficiency so closely resembled eczema, it seemed an obvious step to measure the amounts of fatty acids in the blood of children with atopic eczema. This was done in 1933 by the American paediatrician Arild E. Hansen, who found that children with eczema had lower levels of unsaturated fatty acids in their blood than children without eczema. Hansen and other dermatologists therefore began to treat their eczema patients with dietary supplements of vegetable oils. Some were convinced that this treatment was effective; some were not. Later, more careful studies of the levels of essential fatty acids in the blood of eczema patients showed that normally nourished people do not have a deficiency of these fatty acids. In retrospect, it seems possible that some of the eczematous children checked in the 1930s were undernourished, and that this was the reason for the low fatty acid levels.

This was not the end of the story, however. More recent biochemical research showed that fatty acids had other functions beyond keeping us warm and healthy. In the 1960s and 1970s a new and important family of hormones was discovered. Its members were the eicosanoids and they were all produced from fatty acids. They include the prostaglandins and the leukotrienes which have been found to be of basic importance in many body functions. Prostaglandins are known to be involved in skin inflammation in eczema and are among the substances released by the mast cells and the eosinophils when they degranulate.

This discovery led to the idea that it might be possible, by changing the proportions of dietary fats, to alter the kind of prostaglandins and leukotrienes produced to types that were less liable to damage the skin and thus relieve the severity of eczema. There is a considerable range of prostaglandins with a wide range of properties. One source of dietary fat thought possibly capable of doing this was evening primrose oil. This oil is rich in gamma-linolenic acid. It is often called gamolenic acid and is sold in Britain under the trade names of Epogam, Efamast and Efamol Marine. From the late 1970s onwards many trials of the effectiveness of this substance in eczema followed and were reported in most of the major medical and dermatological journals. Most of these reports indicated at least some measure of success and many doctors were convinced that this was a useful treatment. Proprietary forms of the oil were added to the list of drugs that could be prescribed on the National Health Service.

There were, however, many critics, especially of the validity of these trials and of the form that they took. A paper in the *Lancet* in November 1989 criticized some unjustified claims by drug companies. This paper did not mention evening primrose oil, but it sparked off a controversy between some hospital dermatologists and doctors working for a drug firm promoting Epogam for eczema. The hospital doctors took the view that none of the trials of evening primrose oil had proved its efficacy; the manufacturer's doctors denied this and insisted that the evidence in favour of the drug was conclusive. This argument ran for several issues of the *Lancet* and brought out some interesting points, in particular the ease with which such trials can produce misleading results. The doctors from the drug company fought back valiantly and, among other telling points, commented that among the seven top-selling drugs used to treat atopic eczema in Britain, evening primrose oil was the only one that had been tested in double-blind, placebo-controlled trials. Those that had not been tested in this way included several steroid preparations for local use.

After this letter, the editor of the *Lancet* seems to have decided that the matter had been sufficiently aired and we were left wondering what was the truth of it all. Since then the situation in the medical press has been fairly quiet with only occasional references to evening primrose oil. In June 1993, however, a paper appeared in the *Lancet* describing a carefully organized double-blind, placebo-controlled trial of evening primrose oil involving 123 patients with atopic eczema and lasting for 16 weeks. The results were assessed by keeping scores of severity both by the doctors and by the patients themselves. The scoring system recorded changes, if any, in redness, dryness, cracking, scaliness and the effects of scratching (excoriation). They also recorded whether and how the requirement for local steroid applications changed. Sadly, the results were entirely negative. There was no clear evidence that evening primrose oil helped in any way.

This result was in agreement with the largest previous study of evening primrose oil in atopic eczema, which was published in the *Journal of the American Academy of Dermatology* in 1985. This study of 154 patients also showed no benefit from evening primrose oil.

The current view of the experts seems to be veering away from belief in the efficacy of evening primrose oil in eczema and other conditions. In a leading article in the *British Medical Journal* in October 1994, a clinical epidemiologist from the University of Amsterdam concluded that although evening primrose oil was an interesting substance there was little justification for its use in many of the conditions for which it was claimed to be effective. This was not to say that the drug was useless but that none of the trials had proved conclusively that it was useful. Interestingly, in the dosage commonly recommended, the oil contains a megadose of vitamin E. The research evidence for the value of vitamin E as an antioxidant effective against disease-producing agencies known as free radicals is becoming increasingly convincing.

After all that, you are probably going to have to make up your own mind about evening primrose oil. At least it is harmless.

Traditional Chinese remedies

In contrast to the frequently expressed scepticism about evening primrose oil, there is a surprising amount of acceptance, even among dermatologists, of certain traditional Chinese remedies for eczema. As one senior consultant in paediatric dermatology put it: 'Chinese medicines have produced impressive responses in cases of atopic eczema that have proved resistant to conventional treatment'.

Characteristics of traditional Chinese medicine

It is a mistake to assume that a medical remedy must be effective because it is old and comes from an unfamiliar culture. Much of traditional Chinese medicine is based on very shaky logic. Drugs are used, in balanced formulations, to counter effects which are apparent to the patient. 'Cool' drugs, such as extracts of mint and chrysanthemum, are used for 'hot' disorders such as fevers. Sweet herbs deal with 'sour' symptoms, such as dyspepsia, while sour preparations are given for their astringent or 'solidifying' effect. Disease is regarded as an imbalance between the forces of Yin (excess) and Yang (deficiency), and recovery, practitioners believe, is to be obtained by correcting the balance.

Every town in the world with any major Chinese population has its traditional medicine shops stocked with an amazing variety of herbs, animal parts and minerals purporting to have medicinal value. Most of the Chinese population relies on these old remedies and the shops are often crowded. In Britain there are more than 600 Chinese medicine clinics offering traditional remedies.

In connection with eczema it is important to recognize what is

73

meant by the word 'remedy'. Systems of medicine that are not scientific in the Western sense, including much of traditional Chinese medicine, are commonly concerned with abolishing symptoms and signs. Scientific medicine always regards symptoms and signs as an indication of an underlying disease process and tries, if it can, to find that process and eliminate it. Thus, it is considered bad medicine simply to 'treat symptoms' as is done in Chinese medicine. A true remedy is one which cures the condition that is causing the symptom.

When an underlying cause cannot be found, however, it is, of course, legitimate and proper to do whatever is possible to relieve the patient of the distress of the symptoms. This is done so long as the symptomatic treatment does not endanger the patient or reduce the chances of finding a diagnosis. Regrettably, none of the treatments for eczema, whether Chinese or Western, can be regarded as definitive cures for eczema in the sense that the condition is eliminated and will not recur. So, if Chinese medicines can be shown to relieve the features of eczema, even for a time, and if they can be shown to be safe, then there can be no reason not to use them and be grateful.

What are the Chinese eczema remedies?

The remedy that has been found effective in controlling itching and producing a noticeable improvement in the skin condition of children with atopic eczema consists of a tea made from herbs. These herbs are listed in traditional Chinese drug manuals (pharmacopoeias) and the botanical names include *Caulis akebiae, Potentilla chinensis, Tribulus terrestris, Rehmannia glutinosa, Glycyrrhiza uralensis, Paeonia lactiflora, Paeonia rubra, Akebia clematidis, Dictamnus dasycarpus, Lophatherum gracile* and *Schizonepeta tenuifolia*. With the exception of *Glycyrrhiza* (liquorice) these herbs are not to be found in modern Western pharmacopoeias. Liquorice is, of course, well known in the West but you may not be aware that it contains glycyrrhetinic acid – a drug that relieves inflammation and also increases the effect of the steroid hydrocortisone when both are locally applied.

Usually about ten of these herbs are boiled in water, and the extracts mixed in various proportions. Each prescription is adjusted according to the perceived need of each individual patient. Analytic chemical studies at the London School of Pharmacy have isolated more than 30 pure chemical substances from these herbs.

Do they work?

Several trials of Chinese herbal remedies in atopic eczema have apparently shown useful effect. Not all of these trials have been designed and conducted with the standards of care necessary to avoid misleading or statistically unconvincing results. Some, however, have been of a high standard.

One of the most impressive was reported in the *Lancet* in July, 1992. This trial was done on 40 patients aged 16 to 65, each with a long history of extensive atopic eczema that had resisted conventional medical treatment. All of them had eczema covering at least 20 per cent of the body area. The patients were divided randomly into two groups. One group was given a tea of ten herbs previously found to be effective in eczema; the other group was given a placebo mixture with a similar taste and smell to the trial mixture but containing none of the Chinese herbs. After two months, the treatment was stopped for four weeks and the treatments were then switched, so that those who had been having the herb tea now had the placebo, and vice versa. The trial then continued for a further two months. The four-week interval before the switch-over was to ensure that any effective drugs persisting in the patients' bodies would have gone.

At no time during the trial did any of the patients know whether they were taking the placebo or the active treatment. The doctors conducting the trial were also unaware of which preparation was which. No side effects were noted during the trial, but many of the patients reported that both of the teas tasted really horrible.

The patients' bodies were charted into 20 roughly equal areas and scoring was done on each of these. Criteria used were redness and extent of surface changes as shown by blistering, scaling, lichenification (see chapter 1) and the effects of scratching (excoriation). So far as area affected in each of the 20 zones was concerned, a score of 0 was given if the area was unaffected; 1 was given if less than one third was affected; 2 if the area affected was between one third and two thirds; and 3 if more than two thirds were affected. These were then averaged up to give a whole body score. Severity, for each of the 20 areas, was also assessed on a score of 0 to 3 and these were added together. The final score was obtained by multiplying the sum of the severity scores with the area scores, giving a maximum score of 180.

The outcome was surprisingly good. For redness, patients taking the herb tea had an average score, at the end of the trial period, of 12.6; those taking the placebo averaged 113. For area damaged, patients taking the herb tea had an average score 11.3; those taking the placebo averaged 111. The results were also judged by the patients themselves. Of the 24 patients who expressed a preference, 20 opted for the herb tea and 4 for the placebo.

Are Chinese remedies safe?

The big problem, here, is that we simply don't know how much of the active ingredient there is in a particular medicine. This brings up the question of standardization. Western pharmacologists are very much aware that the effect of most drugs varies with the dose and that nearly all active drugs are dangerous if too much is taken. For this reason, when drugs are prepared from plants in the West, considerable trouble is taken to ensure that a standard dose of the drug contains a known amount of the effective substance. The simplest way to ensure this is to extract the active ingredient and purify it so that one is dealing with a single substance. It is then necessary only to weigh it to know how much is being given. If this is impossible, the drug may have to be standardized by actually testing the effect of the particular sample in various ways. This can sometimes be difficult.

Unfortunately, retailers of the Chinese remedies simply take various quantities of the dried herbs and make up their concoctions. This rough and ready way of preparing a medicine is not considered acceptable, by Western standards, especially if the herbs contain potentially dangerous substances. There are several ways in which the amounts of the active ingredient might vary widely. Plants synthesize biochemicals to different extents at different stages in their growth cycles. They may also produce different amounts if grown in different places with differing soil mineral content. Quite apart from these factors, it would still be possible to extract varying amounts by a lack of standardization in the methods used to make the decoction.

Some, for instance, might be boiled for longer periods than others. It is even possible that different mixtures of herbs might affect the amount of a particular ingredient appearing in the final liquid.

That these are no mere theoretical concerns is shown by the fact that the analysis of a dozen samples of the same Chinese herb bought in London yielded amounts of the active ingredient ranging from 0.01 per cent to 4.5 per cent. This is a range of 450 to 1 and is worrying. Such a range would never be considered acceptable for any Western drug taken by mouth and indicates that patients may be getting a widely varying dosage. Reports have appeared in the *British Medical Journal*, the *Lancet*, the *Journal of Clinical Gastroenterology* and other medical journals of liver damage caused by Chinese herbal remedies. There are even reports of a few cases of fatal hepatitis strongly suspected of having been caused by Chinese herb remedies. In one of these, the herb *Teucrium chamaedrys* (wild germander) was deemed to be the probable cause of death. Germander is known from other cases to cause liver damage. In other cases, the responsible herb was not identified.

It would be unfair to imply that all Chinese herbal practitioners are indifferent to these dangers. Some of the larger Chinese clinics have facilities for biochemical screening and for tests that can detect such effects as liver damage. It would also be unfair to suggest that these concerns apply only to Chinese remedies. Western doctors have for some time been worried about herbal remedies in general, and many reports have been published describing cases of illness and death caused by these.

Here is a case history of a child treated with Chinese herbal tea.

CASE HISTORY
Dorothy's eczema showed a remarkably good response to a Chinese herbal remedy. Unfortunately, there was a major snag . . .

PERSONAL DETAILS
Name Dorothy Baltimore
Age 9
Occupation Schoolgirl
Family No siblings; parents alive and well.

MEDICAL BACKGROUND

Dorothy first developed eczema at the age of three months and had suffered moderately severely ever since. The case was typical. At first it had affected mainly her face and head and had spared her limbs. Later, the scaliness and redness had cleared from her face and had affected the flexures of her knees and elbows and the adjoining areas of the limbs.

She had had all the usual local remedies with little useful effect and her parents had become increasingly distressed. They had told the doctor that they felt sure something else could be done to restore normality to their daughter's skin.

THE PRESENT COMPLAINT

Mrs Baltimore brought Dorothy to the doctor because, for over two weeks, the girl had been complaining of pain in the centre of her tummy, sickness and a worrying total loss of appetite.

THE EXAMINATION

The first thing the doctor notices is that Dorothy's skin, and the whites of her eyes, show a slight but definite yellow tinge. Mrs Baltimore has not mentioned this but, when it is drawn to her notice, she says that for a day or two she has thought that the skin might be discoloured. The doctor explains that this is jaundice and asks Dorothy if she has noticed anything unusual when she goes to the toilet. At first, Dorothy denies that there has been anything strange, but, on prompting, says that her poos are a very peculiar colour – a sort of whitish-grey, like the clay they use in handicrafts at school.

The doctor gets Dorothy to lie down on the examination couch and gently feels her tummy. He finds that her liver is enlarged and slightly tender. He asks Mrs Baltimore whether the family has been abroad recently. Mrs Baltimore says 'No'. He also confirms that Dorothy has had no blood transfusions or anaesthetics.

Dorothy is very brave when the doctor tells her that he must take some blood from her arm. She looks away as he does it and feels only a brief sharp pricking sensation. Arrangements are made to see her again in two weeks' time. Meanwhile Dorothy is to stay quietly at home and to wash very carefully after using the toilet.

THE SECOND CONSULTATION

When the doctor sees Dorothy again he tells Mrs Baltimore that Dorothy has hepatitis. The jaundice is due to the fact that the inflamed liver is no longer able to excrete the coloured breakdown products of red blood cell destruction into the bowel. As a result the stools are pale and the pigment accumulating in her blood colours the skin. He is a little puzzled, however, as there are no indications that the condition is infective. Again he questions the mother about any unusual circumstances.

This time it is Dorothy who speaks up. 'I think it's that horrible Chinese medicine,' she says.

The doctor questions Mrs Baltimore who admits, with some embarrassment, that they have been seeing a Chinese practitioner who has been treating Dorothy's eczema and getting very good results. The doctor looks thoughtful then says that there have been reports of liver damage from Chinese eczema remedies. He says that he cannot be sure that this is the cause of Dorothy's hepatitis, but insists that the risk is too great to take. He strongly advises that Dorothy should stop taking the medicine immediately.

THE FOLLOW-UP

Dorothy's parents accept this advice and stop the concoction. Over the course of the next two months the jaundice slowly fades and Dorothy's liver returns to its normal size. The blood tests of liver function also return to normal.

Unfortunately, as this happens, Dorothy's eczema gets much worse and her parents, although aware of the risks, decide to resume the Chinese medicine. At the same time, the doctor arranges for monitoring of the liver function by blood tests. After a month's treatment, although Dorothy feels fine, the tests show early abnormalities of liver function. In addition, her liver can once more be felt below the rib margin, indicating that it has again become enlarged.

This time the doctor is particularly firm. If Dorothy continues to take the concoction he cannot be responsible for the consequences. Regretfully, the parents agree to stop it. Over the course of several months, Dorothy's eczema gradually settles to much about the state it was in before she started taking the herbal treatment.

Current medical opinion on Chinese herbal medicines

The pharmacology of Chinese herbal remedies is still largely unknown. It is, however, almost certainly a mistake to assume that these herbs contain some magic remedy unknown to Western science. What is far more likely is that some of them contain chemicals that can act at various cell receptors to modify the action of the cells or the action of existing hormones on them. Some may influence the action of the immune system in various ways. These are the kind of ways in which some of our established Western drugs work.

Already research has shown that some of the Chinese herbal ingredients have sedative properties; some actually control pain; and some are active against inflammation. But we already have drugs with these properties – drugs which are known to be safe. It would, however, be a mistake to dismiss Chinese herbal remedies. Most experts now agree that a good deal of further research is needed to show whether the Chinese pharmacopoeia contains substances substantially better for treating eczema than existing drugs while, at the same time, being safe. It is, however, not beyond the bounds of possibility that such research might reveal a drug which, purified and standardized, could become as important in eczema as penicillin was in bacterial infection.

Meantime there have been calls for the scrupulous standardization of these remedies so that the doses given are known.

10
Avoiding Eczema

There is much to be done to reduce the likelihood of episodes of eczema or to cut down its severity. Avoidance is, of course, based on knowledge of precipitating factors and on the possibility of ensuring that they do not gain access to the body. This can sometimes be very difficult as the following case history illustrates.

CASE HISTORY
Owen's severe eczema was known to be related to food intolerance. This had been proved by proper laboratory tests. But the management of this unfortunate state of affairs raised further problems . . .

PERSONAL DETAILS
Name Owen Fields
Age 3 years 7 months
Occupation N/A
Family No siblings; mother has asthma.

MEDICAL BACKGROUND
Owen first developed atopic eczema at the age of six months and this had responded poorly to conventional local treatment with softening ointments and local steroids. Recently, the family have moved to this area and have immediately registered for medical care.

THE MEDICAL CONSULTATION
Owen's doctor is distressed to find that more than 40 per cent of his whole body surface is affected by eczema. The unfortunate child is tortured by itching and he has so damaged his skin by scratching that his distracted parents have had to restrain him. Questioning reveals that, in addition to the eczema, Owen often suffers severe attacks of hives brought on by eating fish, eggs or split peas. The doctor recognizes that the eczema is related to this strong allergic

element. She also appreciates that this is a particularly difficult and worrying case and decides that specialist attention is needed. She therefore arranges for Owen to be seen at a paediatric department where, she knows, there are physicians with a particular interest in such problems.

MANAGEMENT IN PAEDIATRIC OUTPATIENTS

The specialist takes a detailed history of Owen's skin problems. It is immediately apparent that the allergic element is of overwhelming importance in Owen's eczema. Investigation indicates that the skin upset is related to house dust mites, timothy grass, cats and dogs. It is also clear that Owen's eczema always gets significantly worse after he has eaten wheat, codfish, eggs, tomatoes, blackcurrants or strawberries or has drunk cow's milk. Full investigation is undertaken.

Tests of Owen's IgE levels show the quite extraordinary figure of 68,000 nanograms per millilitre. The normal for a child of his age is less than 42 nanograms. In view of these findings and the severity of the eczema the specialists decide to put him, for a time, on a diet limited to potato, rice, Rice Crispies, brussels sprouts and lamb. Soon after starting on this restricted diet, Owen's eczema improves dramatically.

This is encouraging, but it is necessary to find other foods he can safely take so as to extend the range of his diet. To this end, single foods are re-introduced one at a time, at weekly intervals. In the course of this trial it is found that milk, casein hydrolysate milk formulas and soya milk all cause intolerance. This is unfortunate as it is apparent that Owen's restricted diet will be dangerously low in calcium. To remedy this, Owen is prescribed calcium tablets to be taken once a day.

After he has taken only two tablets Owen's eczema gets worse and continues to worsen for six weeks. The tablets are stopped and the eczema improves rapidly. A different calcium preparation is tried and within two days a severe, widespread, itchy red rash appears. This settles when the tablets are stopped. Further trials a few months later produce the same effect. By now the doctors are becoming seriously worried about the deficiencies of calcium in

Owen's diet. Tests show that his intake is only about 13 per cent of the recommended daily allowance. He is now given a powder of pure calcium gluconate and within two days the eczema is much worse. His parents are persuaded to continue with the powder for two weeks but by the end of this time 80 per cent of Owen's body surface is severely inflamed. Within a week of stopping the calcium the flare-up settles. The worried specialists decide that Owen should be admitted to hospital for treatment.

MANAGEMENT IN HOSPITAL

In hospital Owen is given a specially-prepared solution of calcium gluconate by intravenous drip. He is also given vitamin A and D supplements. Unfortunately, his apparent calcium allergy reasserts itself and within three days the itching becomes intense and the drip is stopped. The eczema continues to worsen for a few days, however, but within a week has returned to the state it was in before the infusion was started. Long-acting antihistamine drugs are given and the calcium restarted but regrettably, the effects are the same.

Calcium allergy has not previously been reported. On general principles, also, it seems very unlikely that such a thing could occur. Calcium is such a vital element in the body, and the bones and other tissues contain so much of it that the doctors are not convinced that Owen is actually allergic to this element. Enquiries show that all the preparations of calcium suitable for medical use contain small traces of other substances such as various proteins and fatty acids. And, of course, all calcium-containing foodstuffs contain many other ingredients. It seems likely that the allergy is due to some associated substance.

Owen is allowed home while further enquiries are pursued.

THE FOLLOW-UP

After many distressing trials, a soya-based preparation is found which, to the surprise of everyone, Owen is able to tolerate. This contains plenty of calcium and it is unnecessary for him to have any other source of this important element. Owen is now known to be able to tolerate 33 different foods and can take a modestly varied diet. His eczema is fairly well controlled but is always liable to flare up. For a person as remarkably allergic as he is the situation is as good as could reasonably be expected.

This is, of course, an exceptionally severe case. Very few people suffer as much as Owen has. The case is included mainly to illustrate the unfortunate effect of repeated allergic attacks with the resulting build-up of IgE in the body. Anyone with the kind of IgE levels found in Owen's case may be expected to be very badly affected.

The moral is that every effort should be made to avoid the allergens that promote such increases in the allergy immunoglobulin – IgE.

Preventing eczema

It is of the first importance to reduce or avoid as many as possible of the various factors that trigger episodes of atopic dermatitis. There are many of these trigger factors and they can be divided into two large groups – allergens and non-allergens. In some cases, there is uncertainty as to whether a particular trigger factor is an allergen or not. This distinction is academic; all factors known to bring on eczema or to make it worse should be strenuously avoided.

Allergen triggers are dealt with in chapter 3 and you will see that one of the most important is the house dust mite (see below). Factors that can trigger eczema but are mainly non-allergens are also important and include:

- overheating
- electric blankets
- profuse sweating
- prickly heat with sweat retention
- changes in temperature or humidity
- strongly smelling irritants
- fumes of various kinds
- atmospheric ozone
- smoke pollution

- atmospheric sulphur dioxide
- emotional upset
- psychological stress
- colds and other upper respiratory tract infections
- skin infections
- infections elsewhere in the body
- discharge from the sinuses
- alcohol
- strenuous exertion, especially in cold air
- scratching
- excessive bathing or showering
- rough-textured clothing
- woollen garments
- bleaches
- greasy skin applications.

This list is given as a general contrast to the allergenic substances listed in chapter 3. You should note, however, that some of the substances mentioned here can also act as allergens to which sensitivity can develop. This is especially true of substances that come into contact with the skin. Note, also, that a great many cleaning and washing materials now contain enzymes to serve various purposes. This may be so even if they are not described as 'biological'.

Very small traces of trigger substances can cause eczema or worsen existing eczema. For this reason, clothing should be carefully washed with mild soap powders and thoroughly rinsed before being dried.

Food allergy

This is especially important during the first two years of life. During these early years the commonest allergen responsible for promoting eczema is probably cow's milk. Many cases of infantile eczema have been cured by the elimination of cow's milk and cow's milk products from the diet. Because very small amounts of these substances can cause problems, this may be more difficult than is imagined. There are several kinds of milk-free formulas for babies:

- soya-based formulas (Isomil, Ostersoy, Wysoy, Nutrilon Soya or Prosobee);
- casein hydrolysates (Pregestimil, Nutramigen or Lofenalac);
- whey hydrolysates (Alfare Nestlé);
- comminuted chicken formula.

Although the hydrolysates are made from cow's milk this is treated with enzymes so that the milk protein is partially broken down to simple molecules that are less likely to be allergenic. Whey hydrolysates, which are made from the liquid whey that separates from the curds when the milk is curdled with rennin, are less likely to be allergenic than casein hydrolysates.

Surprisingly, babies' eczema can be made significantly worse by cow's milk and other allergens derived from the mother's milk during breast feeding. Two interesting studies on this were reported in the *British Medical Journal* in July 1986. These were double-blind, cross-over trials involving 37 breast-fed infants with eczema. In the cases of six of the babies, the eczema improved when the mothers eliminated cow's milk and eggs from their own diets. Significantly, the eczema got worse again when the mothers started taking milk and eggs again.

In older people, food allergy is not a common cause of eczema but, as we have seen, when it does occur, it can be very serious. In general, however, dietary restrictions are seldom needed unless there are clear indications that a particular food can be implicated in causing worsening of the eczema. If food allergy is suspected, a skin prick test can be done to narrow the field of investigation. In this test, a small drop of a solution containing an extract of various food substances is placed on the skin and a small prick is made with a needle through the drop. A positive result is shown by an obvious raised, red area. Such a result does not prove that a food allergy is causing the eczema. Only about half of those with a positive skin prick reaction to a particular food substance are found to develop skin symptoms after eating the food concerned.

Certain foods are more likely to promote eczema than others. It is probably wise, in atopic families, to avoid giving babies such foods altogether for the first six months of life or even for the first year. This is especially so if there are brothers or sisters who have developed eczema. Foods that are best avoided are:

- eggs
- cow's milk
- wheat
- fish
- chocolate
- nuts, especially peanuts
- yeast
- oranges.

It is easy to overestimate the importance of food allergy in general, and its role in eczema in particular. Even within the medical profession there has been a good deal of controversy. The arguments have not been helped by the activities and claims of a number of practitioners of alternative medicine. A good deal of what is written in the popular press about food allergy is exaggerated, inaccurate or just plain nonsense.

House dust mites

One of the most important provocative factors of atopic eczema is the allergen produced by the house dust mite *Dermatophagoides pteronyssinus*. This microscopic creature, which lives on human skin scales and thrives in moist atmospheres, is present in enormous numbers in most households, especially in bedrooms. Large numbers of mites are also found in children's soft toys. In order to digest human keratin, the mites' DNA code creates a gene to produce an enzyme that can break down this protein. The enzyme is, of course, present in the intestines of the mites and the droppings of the animals are covered with it. This enzyme is the actual allergen that causes the trouble.

What to do about house dust mites

Thorough vacuum cleaning of a bedroom or sitting room can immediately reduce the mite population by 70 per cent. Unfortunately, these little creatures breed very rapidly and the population will have returned to the previous level within a week. So frequent hoovering is needed if it is to be really effective. Dust mite excreta are highly allergenic and are an important cause of repeated episodes of eczema. Don't forget, however, that vacuum cleaning causes mite faeces to become airborne, so the eczema sufferer must be well out of the way, otherwise the allergen will be inhaled. It doesn't really matter how the enzyme gets into the body; it will readily produce IgE if inhaled.

Few of the old-fashioned cloth bag vacuum cleaners are still in use and those which use tough, disposable paper bags are more efficient in retaining dust mite droppings. But these particles are very small indeed and can readily get through with the expelled air. They are more likely to be trapped if the bag has already been used for a while so that the air has to pass through a thick layer of fluff and dust. For this reason bedrooms should not be the first rooms to be vacuum cleaned immediately after a bag is changed.

Miticides are chemicals that can kill house dust mites, and are worth considering. They include tannic acid, crotamiton and benzyl benzoate. Some people treat their carpets with these. Unfortunately, benzyl benzoate can cause severe skin irritation, which is the last thing eczema sufferers need. It can also damage the eyes. So you must be careful not to overdo the use of these miticide substances. Probably the most effective measure against mites is to deprive them of their favourite habitat – cotton or linen sheets, pillow-slips, duvet covers and mattresses. If these are enclosed in polythene or nylon bags the mites will have a hard time of it. Do be very careful, however, with children's bedding, and ensure that there is no possibility of a plastic bag coming loose and causing suffocation. Bedding should also be washed frequently at a high temperature setting of the washing machine. This will help to keep down the mite population.

Children's soft toys are also common breeding grounds for house dust mites. Teddy bears, for instance, can soon become heavily infested and provide a continuing and unsuspected source of allergen. The best solution, in this case, is a weekly stay in the freezer. The water in the mites freezes and kills them so that no more allergenic enzyme is released. House dust mites are also very sensitive to reduced atmospheric humidity. Experience has shown that people with severe atopic eczema are often greatly improved during a spell in an Alpine region at an altitude above 1000 metres. At such altitudes, the air is so dry that house dust mites cannot survive.

11

Glossary

acute Short, sharp and quickly over. Acute conditions usually start abruptly, last for a few days and then either settle or become persistent and long-lasting (chronic). Eczema is a chronic condition but may often have acute flare-ups. The term is derived from the Latin *acutus*, meaning 'sharp'.

acyclovir A drug highly active against the Herpes simplex virus and against the closely similar varicella-zoster virus which causes chickenpox and shingles. Early treatment with the drug, taken by mouth, can greatly reduce the severity of shingles. See also **Kaposi's varicelliform eruption**. A trade name is Zovirax.

adenopathy Any inflammation, abnormal enlargement or other disorder of lymph nodes. The term literally means any disease of glands, and lymph nodes are not glands, but common usage restricts the meaning to lymph node disease or affection. Adenopathy in the nodes draining an eczematous area of skin implies that the condition has become secondarily infected, and is a sign that treatment is urgently needed.

allergen Any substance capable of producing an allergic reaction in a person after contacting or entering the body. To act, an allergen must at least pass through the surface layers of cells of the epidermis. See chapters 2 and 3.

allergic dermatitis Inflammation of the skin following contact with any substance to which the person is allergic. See chapters 3 and 5.

allergy Hypersensitivity to body contact with a foreign substance (an **allergen**), especially grass or tree pollens, foods, dust, mites or certain metals such as nickel. The effect may take several forms, including weals (**urticaria**), **dermatitis**, **asthma** or hay fever (allergic rhinitis). An allergic response implies that there has been a prior contact with the allergen during which the immunological processes leading to the hypersensitivity have occurred. Susceptibility to allergy is often of genetic origin. This is called **atopy** and is a principal cause of eczema. The term derives from the Greek *allos*, 'other' and *ergon*, 'work'.

antibiotic drugs An extensive range of drugs able to kill or prevent reproduction of bacteria in the body, without killing the patient. Antibiotics were originally derived from cultures of living organisms, such as fungi or bacteria, but today many are chemically synthesized. The antibiotics have enormously extended the scope and effectiveness of medical therapy against bacterial infection, but have not succeeded in eliminating any bacterial diseases. In eczema, antibiotics are used to treat or to prevent secondary infection. They have no part to play in the management of the underlying processes that cause atopic eczema, unless the eczema is caused by allergy to bacterial bodies.

antibody A protein substance, called an immunoglobulin, produced by the B group of lymphocytes in response to the presence of an **antigen**. An appropriate B lymphocyte is selected from the existing repertoire. This then produces a clone of plasma cells each capable of synthesizing large numbers of specific antibodies to combat the infection. The B cells also produce memory cells. Subsequent infection with the same antigen prompts the memory cells to clone plasma cells and produce the correct antibodies without further delay. This is an important way in which infection results in subsequent immunity. Antibodies are able to neutralize antigens or render them susceptible to destruction by phagocytes in the body. A particular antibody class – IgE – is implicated in the production of atopic eczema.

antigen Any substance, organism or foreign material recognized by the immune system of the body as being 'non-self', which will provoke the production of a specific **antibody**. Antigens include infective viruses, bacteria and fungi, pollen grains, house dust mite droppings and donor tissue. Antigens that cause allergy are called **allergens**.

antihistamine One of a group of drugs which act against histamine – a powerful and highly irritant agent released in the body by **mast cells**, after contact with certain **allergens**. Antihistamine drugs have a minor but important part to play in the management of eczema. This is because they can relieve the itching that is such an important feature of the condition. In children they are also useful in promoting sleep disturbed by itching. There are many antihistamine drugs. They include diphenhydramine (Benadryl), chlorpheniramine (Piriton), terfenadine (Triludan), promethazine (Phenergan), mepyramine (Anthisan), cyproheptadine (Periactin), mequitazine (Primalan) and phenindamine (Thephorin).

anti-inflammatory Acting against inflammation. The most important and effective anti-inflammatory drugs are the **corticosteroids-** ('steroids'). These are widely used in the treatment of eczema.

asthma A disease in which the circular smooth muscles of the branching air tubes of the lungs are liable to go into a state of spasm so that they are narrowed and the passage of air is impeded. The bronchospasm may be induced by a variety of stimuli, but sensitivity to an allergy-causing substance (**allergen**) is amongst the commonest. Allergic asthma is related to atopic eczema in that both share essentially the same causation and trigger factors. Many people have both.

atopic eczema A common form of dermatitis caused by allergy to an **allergen** operating at a site which may be remote from that at which the allergen first contacts the body. Thus inhaled house dust mite droppings may cause the skin reactions known as eczema. Atopic eczema is a hereditary condition caused by genes that affect the sites at which antibodies of the class IgE attach themselves to cell walls. See also **atopy**.

atopy An inherited tendency in which environmental factors can cause the person concerned to develop eczema, asthma or hay fever. Atopy is a hypersensitivity state associated with immunoglobulin E (IgE). A gene for atopy has been identified and others are expected to be found in due course. The term is derived from the Greek *a*, 'not' and *topos*, 'a place'.

contact dermatitis Skin inflammation caused by an allergic reaction to a substance that has been in contact with the skin. See chapter 5.

contact eczema See **contact dermatitis**.

corticosteroids See **steroid drugs**.

dermatitis Inflammation of the skin from any cause. Dermatitis is not a specific disease, but any one of a large range of inflammatory disorders featuring redness, blister formation, swelling, weeping, crusting and itching. See chapter 5.

dermatology The study of the skin and its disorders and their relationship to medical conditions in general.

desquamation Shedding, peeling or scaling of skin.

excoriation Immediate physical damage caused by scratching.

eczema herpeticum See **Kaposi's varicelliform eruption**.

erythema Redness of the skin from widening (dilatation) of the small skin blood vessels. This may result from one of a very large number of causes such as blushing, rosacea, permanent widening (ectasia) of blood vessels, inflammation and rashes (exanthemata).

exfoliation Shedding of cells from a surface, such as the skin. In the dangerous condition of exfoliative dermatitis, much of the surface of the skin peels off or is shed. The term comes from the Latin *ex-* meaning 'off', and *folium*, 'leaf'.

exfoliative dermatitis See **exfoliation**.

herpes viruses A group of viruses that includes the Herpes simplex virus, types I and II, causing, respectively, 'cold sores' and venereal herpes, the Herpes zoster virus that causes chickenpox and shingles, the Epstein Barr virus that causes glandular fever (infective mononucleosis) and the cytomegalovirus that affects people with immunodeficiency disorders. Herpes simplex virus infection of skin damaged by eczema can be a serious complication (see **Kaposi's varicelliform eruption**). From the Greek *herpein*, 'to creep'.

hyperkeratosis Undue thickening of the outer layer of the skin so that a dense horny layer, such as a corn or callosity, results. This is a normal and essentially protective response to local pressure. Hyperkeratosis is a feature of long-term (chronic) eczema and may also occur as an inherited disorder of the palms and the soles, or as the disorder **ichthyosis**.

ichthyosis A fish-scale-like disorder of the skin, usually hereditary and present from birth. The outer layer of the skin is thickened and rough and is unable to retain water so that it tends to dry out. Protective and waterproof barrier creams are used.

infantile eczema Atopic dermatitis affecting young children. This is one of the several alternative terms for the disorder.

infective eczema Eczema that had been complicated by secondary infection of the skin by bacteria, viruses or fungi.

intertrigo Dermatitis that occurs in areas of skin that remain constantly in contact with each other, especially in the groins and armpits. Intertrigo affects obese people, mostly in hot climates.

Kaposi's varicelliform eruption A widespread secondary infection of eczematous skin with Herpes simplex or other viruses. This is a serious complication that may spread to involve the central nervous system with possible fatal consequences. Because of the danger of causing this condition, people with cold sores must keep well away from children and others with eczema. Smallpox has been eradicated so, happily, there is no longer any justification for vaccination with vaccinia viruses. Also known as eczema herpeticum.

lichenification Hardened and thickened skin epidermis caused by abnormally persistent scratching. This is usually a response to some long-term (chronic) skin condition such as eczema but may be the result of mental agitation and the establishment of a scratch-itch-scratch-itch vicious cycle. Lichenification soon disappears if scratching can be avoided.

maculopapular Pertaining to small, circumscribed, usually discoloured, slightly raised spots on the skin.

mast cell A tissue cell found in large numbers in the skin and mucous membranes and in the lymphatic system. The mast cell plays a central part in atopic eczema. It contains numerous granules – collections of powerfully irritating chemical substances. In people with allergies, the antibody IgE remains attached to specific receptors on the surface of the mast cells. When the substance causing the allergy (the **allergen**) contacts the IgE, the mast cell is triggered to release these substances and the result is the range of allergic symptoms and signs, including eczema.

nanogram One thousand-millionth of a gram (Greek *nanos*, 'dwarf').

papule Any small, well-defined, solid skin elevation. Papules are usually less than 1 centimetre in diameter and may be smooth or warty. From the Latin *papula*, 'pimple'.

pruritus Itching. The term is often linked with a word that indicates the site, as in pruritus ani or pruritus vulvae. Pruritus is the cardinal symptom of eczema and is such a common feature that doctors will hesitate to make the diagnosis without it. Note that the word should not be spelled 'pruritis', which implies inflammation. It derives from the Latin *prurire*, meaning 'to itch'.

rash Any inflammatory skin eruption of reasonable extent and of whatever cause.

RAST The radio-allergo-sorbent test. This is a test for specific types of immunoglobulin, class E (IgE) used to determine to which particular substance or substances a person is allergic. The IgE class contains a very large number of different immunoglobulins, each being specific for a particular allergen such as the enzymes on house dust mite droppings, various animal product allergens or food allergens. The RAST can identify the particular IgE and hence the allergen.

spongiosis The collection of numerous tiny droplets of fluid in the skin, especially in the epidermis. Oedema of the skin.

steroid drugs A large group of drugs that are derived from, resemble, or simulate the actions of, the natural **corticosteroids** or the male sex hormones of the body. Steroids are probably the most important drugs in the treatment of eczema.

urticaria An allergic skin condition featuring itchy, raised, pink areas surrounded by pale skin. These patches persist for periods of half an hour to several days and then resolve. Urticaria may result from sunlight, cold, food or drug allergy, insect bites, scabies, jelly-fish stings or contact with plants. Treatment is with antihistamine drugs or corticosteroids. Also known popularly as nettle rash or hives.

vesicle Any small blister. From the Latin *vesiculum*, 'small bladder or bag'.

Useful Addresses

The National Eczema Society,
Tavistock House North,
Tavistock Square,
London WC1H 9SR
Tel: 0171 388 4097

British Association of Dermatologists,
3 St Andrew's Place,
London NW1 4LB
Tel: 0171 935 8576

British Allergy Foundation,
St Bartholomew's Hospital,
West Smithfield,
London EC1A 7BE
Tel: 0171 600 6127

British Association for Early Childhood,
111 City View,
Bethnal Green Road,
London E2 9QH
Tel: 0171 739 7594

Health and Safety Executive,
Baynards House,
Chepstow Place,
London W2 4TF
Tel: 0171 243 6000

Department of Health,
Health Information Services
Tel: Freephone 0800 66 55 44

The American Academy of Allergy and Immunology,
611 East Wells Street,
Milwaukee, Wisconsin 53202

The American College of Allergy,
800 East Northwest Highway,
Suite 1080,
Palatine, Illinois 60067

The National Institute of Allergy and Infectious Diseases,
Building 31, Room 7A33,
Bethesda, Maryland 20892

The National Allergy and Asthma Association,
3554 Chain Bridge Road, Suite 200,
Fairfax, Virginia 22030

The Asthma and Allergy Foundation of America,
1125 15th Street NW, Suite 502,
Washington DC 20005

Further reading

Atopic eczema

Dermatology in Practice (May/ June 1989), p. 18

Atopic eczema management

Lancet (28 May 1994), pp. 1338, 1342

Chinese herbal remedies for eczema

British Journal of Hospital Medicine (16 June 1993), p. 71

Chinese medicines for eczema

British Medical Journal (19 February 1994), p. 489

Chinese herbal remedies

Lancet (4 July 1992), p. 13

Eczema and diet

British Medical Journal (3 December 1988), p. 1458

Atopic dermatitis

British Journal of Hospital Medicine (19 October 1994), p. 409

Atopic dermatitis

Journal of the American Medical Association (25 November 1992), p. 2862

Oral steroids for eczema

Journal of the American Medical Association (14 October 1993), p. 502

Genetics and atopy

British Medical Journal (23 October 1993), p. 1019

Lancet (25 June 1994), p. 1597

Evening primrose oil

Lancet (7 July 1990), p. 50

Hand eczema

Dermatology in Practice (April/ May 1988), p. 30

Diet and atopic eczema

British Medical Journal (3 December 1988), p. 1458

Food intolerance

New Scientist (8 July 1989), p. 45

Evening primrose oil

British Medical Journal (1 October 1994), p. 824

Index

antihistamine drugs 62
atopic eczema: changes with
    age 31; features of 31;
    symptoms of 33
atopy 17; gene for 18; meaning
    of term 16

cell receptors 17, 19
Chinese remedies 73; dangers
    of 76; medical opinion on 80
contact dermatitis 40; common
    causes of 41; from allergy 41;
    from irritants 40
cow's milk dangers 84
cell receptors 17, 19

*Dermatophagoides
    pteronyssinus* 87
dermis 12

eczema: allergen triggers of 27;
    and antibodies 20; and
    asthma 5; avoiding 81; and
    cataract 49; Chinese remedies
    for 73; common sites of 25;
    complications of 47; and food
    allergy 26, 84; frequency of
    4; and hay fever 5; and
    heredity 16; and herpes
    infections 48; and house dust
    mites 87; immune therapy for

64; light therapy for 61;
    meaning of term 3; social
    effects of 55; and temperature
    change 68; treatment of 57;
    worm cure for 22
eczema and dermatitis 1, 4
eczema triggers, avoidance of
    84
Ehrlich, Paul 23
eosinophil cells 22
essential fatty acids 70
evening primrose oil 69
exfoliative dermatitis 49

fats and the skin 70
food allergy 84

goose-pimples 13

hair standing on end 13
histamine 23
Hopkins, Julian 18
house dust mites 87

IgE: levels in blood 21; record
    level of 82; and worms 22
immunoglobulins 20;
    immunoglobulin E 21
inflammation 3
intertrigo 45
itching: cause of 23, 24; control

101